I0799199

The Walking Solution

GET PEOPLE WALKING FOR RESULTS

The Walking Solution

GET PEOPLE WALKING FOR RESULTS

Lee Scott
Michele Stanten

HUMAN KINETICS

Library of Congress Cataloging-in-Publication Data

Names: Scott, Lee, 1969- author. | Stanten, Michele, author.
Title: The walking solution : get people walking for results / Lee Scott, Michele Stanten.
Description: Champaign, Ill. : Human Kinetics, 2020. | Includes bibliographical references and index.
Identifiers: LCCN 2018060587 (print) | LCCN 2019017583 (ebook) | ISBN 9781492591399 (epub) | ISBN 9781492591382 (PDF) | ISBN 9781492575009 (print)
Subjects: LCSH: Walking. | Fitness walking.
Classification: LCC GV502 (ebook) | LCC GV502 .S34 2020 (print) | DDC 613.7/176--dc23
LC record available at https://lccn.loc.gov/2018060587

ISBN: 978-1-4925-7500-9 (print)

Copyright © 2020 by Lee Scott and Michele Stanten

All rights reserved. Except for use in a review, the reproduction or utilization of this work in any form or by any electronic, mechanical, or other means, now known or hereafter invented, including xerography, photocopying, and recording, and in any information storage and retrieval system, is forbidden without the written permission of the publisher.

This publication is written and published to provide accurate and authoritative information relevant to the subject matter presented. It is published and sold with the understanding that the author and publisher are not engaged in rendering legal, medical, or other professional services by reason of their authorship or publication of this work. If medical or other expert assistance is required, the services of a competent professional person should be sought.

The web addresses cited in this text were current as of January 2019, unless otherwise noted.

Senior Acquisitions Editor: Michelle Maloney; **Managing Editor:** Dominique J. Moore; **Copyeditor:** Michelle Horn; **Indexer:** Andrea J. Hepner; **Permissions Manager:** Martha Gullo; **Graphic Designer:** Whitney Milburn; **Cover Designer:** Keri Evans; **Cover Design Associate:** Susan Rothermel Allen; **Photograph (cover):** Keri Evans; **Photographs (interior):** © Human Kinetics; **Photo Asset Manager:** Laura Fitch; **Photo Production Coordinator:** Amy M. Rose; **Photo Production Manager:** Jason Allen; **Senior Art Manager:** Kelly Hendren; **Illustrations:** © Human Kinetics; **Printer:** McNaughton & Gunn, Inc.

Printed in the United States of America 10 9 8 7 6 5 4 3 2 1

The paper in this book is certified under a sustainable forestry program.

Human Kinetics
P.O. Box 5076
Champaign, IL 61825-5076
Website: www.HumanKinetics.com

In the United States, email info@hkusa.com or call 800-747-4457.
In Canada, email info@hkcanada.com.
In the United Kingdom/Europe, email hk@hkeurope.com.

For information about Human Kinetics' coverage in other areas of the world, please visit our website: **www.HumanKinetics.com**

E7459

Tell us what you think!
Human Kinetics would love to hear what we can do to improve the customer experience. Use this QR code to take our brief survey.

CONTENTS

PART V THE BUSINESS OF WALKING

FOREWORD

As a long-time practicing family medicine physician, I have come to realize that exercise is the most powerful medication my patients can take. Not only does it help prevent and treat virtually every chronic disease, but those who take it live longer. In fact, the World Health Organization said that physical inactivity was the fourth leading cause of death around the world, with some 3.3 million attributable deaths per year. Besides the numerous health benefits, my patients who exercise regularly really do look and feel better. In fact, I can usually always tell those who are taking their exercise pill by the way they get on and off the exam table and interact with me. And when I see a senior citizen who is doing all the things they did at 50 when they are 80, without fail, the common denominator seems to be that they engage in regular exercise.

For that reason, I ask every one of my patients about their exercise habits. In fact, we call it an "Exercise Vital Sign," and I want to see my adult patients engaging in at least 150 minutes per week of moderate (or greater) intensity exercise. When I find they are doing this recommended amount of exercise, I simply congratulate them and let them know that I think this is the single best thing they can do for their health. When they are not meeting that 150 minutes per week dose, I always provide them with an exercise prescription. And my default exercise prescription is always walking. There are a variety of reasons that I so often prescribe walking.

First is the fact that walking is accessible. It can be done by all ages, fitness levels, and abilities. It can be done alone or in groups and whether you are at home or traveling. In fact, it is a great way to explore a new place or meet your neighbors when walking at home.

Next, walking is low cost. You don't have to join a gym or buy expensive equipment—just a good pair of shoes and comfortable clothing that keeps you warm in the winter and cool in the summer. That is all you need to get walking.

As a physician, I like the fact that walking is so measurable. I can have my patients use a pedometer, with advice to take 8,000 to 10,000 steps per day. Or I can simply have them time how long they walk using a stop watch, aiming for 30 minutes each day (or three 10-minute walks). Or I can encourage them to walk two miles each day, which takes most adults about 30 minutes to cover when walking at a moderate pace.

I also know that walking is the most common adult activity, with good long-term adherence once people start to do it regularly. And it is the most studied and proven form of physical activity with a robust evidence base proving its benefit.

Finally, I love the fact that walking is cost saving. You don't have to buy a car, gas, bike, or even a bus pass if you walk. And if everyone walked, we know that healthcare costs would be much lower. The planet would also benefit from getting cars off the road and reducing pollution, further adding to the incredible health benefits I have already mentioned.

So, imagine my delight when I learned about this book aimed at promoting walking so that people who need to walk will start and never stop. This book is a how-to guide for those who care about people and want them to be healthy by walking more. It is written by two seasoned fitness professionals who know what works and what doesn't work when it comes to getting people to be more active. Walking is the most powerful drug on the planet, and it is free! The problem is too many people don't understand this fact, and this book can help change that.

Robert Sallis, MD, FAAFP, FACSM
Co-Director, Sports Medicine Fellowship
Kaiser Permanente Medical Center, Fontana, CA;
Advisory Board Chair, Exercise is Medicine Global Health Initiative

PREFACE

Do you fall into one of the following categories?

- A personal trainer trying to attract new clients
- A health club manager looking to increase membership
- A corporate wellness director hoping to curb health care costs
- A yoga studio owner looking to expand offerings
- A health professional eager to help your patients become more active
- A government official interested in making your community healthier

Walking can be your low-cost solution!

Yes, walking! The activity that many think is only for the elderly, obese, or seriously deconditioned is *the* most popular exercise in America. Over 100 million Americans (31 percent of the population) report that they walk for exercise—more than running, cycling, and yoga combined (see graph below). Despite its popularity, walking gets little support and promotion from health and fitness professionals beyond general recommendations. This is a missed opportunity! Fitness and wellness professionals can bring so much to this very accessible activity, making walking a fun and challenging workout.

Year after year, walking outpaces running when it comes to the number of Americans doing it. Here's data for the most recent years (2015, 2016, and 2017). All participation figures are in the thousands.

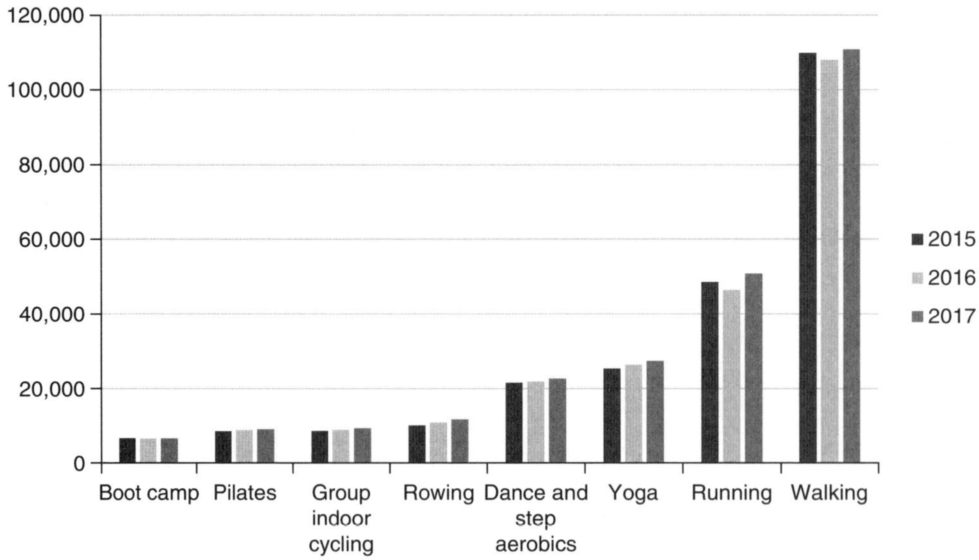

Data from Sport & Fitness Industry Association, *2018 SFIA Sports, Fitness, and Leisure Activities Topline Participation Report* (Jupiter, FL: Sport Marketing Surveys USA, 2018), 16.

Just telling people to walk or even offering basic group walks is not enough. People need walking programs that will keep them interested in walking for fitness.

Michele's Experience

Coaching Tip

A few years ago, a major health insurer in my area opened a retail store and was offering group walks. When I went to check it out one day, I was disappointed when only two other people showed up. Once we started walking, I discovered why. While there was no fee to participate, there was little to no value offered. To say an office staff member led the walk is actually a bit of an exaggeration. She walked with us. There was no leading involved. She didn't offer any advice on walking or other healthy habits. We walked at the pace of the slowest walker. The route was boring. We didn't warm up, cool down, or stretch. There was no encouragement to walk on our own until the next group walk. Sure, there was a bit of group support but not enough to get me, and obviously others, to drive to a location to walk.

The Walking Solution brings the creativity to walking that fitness professionals have been effectively bringing to other forms of exercise for decades. This book will help you create fun, innovative programs that will make it easy for those who are inactive to get moving.

In our experience, walking can be a gateway to an active lifestyle. The success and accomplishment that people feel when they start walking regularly and see improvements can have a snowball effect. It can boost their confidence and encourage them to take a yoga class, join a gym, or hire a trainer. We regularly see people start walking programs, and the next thing you know, they're pulling their bikes out of the garage and going for rides, or they're trying stand-up paddleboarding when they're on vacation. Walking—and especially a walking workout—can give them the confidence to explore other types of physical activity. And those who stick with walking are inspired to take walking to the next level. With a little coaching, they can learn to walk at speeds at which they're burning more calories than if they were jogging at the same pace—and it's easier on their joints. By encouraging them to walk 10Ks, half marathons, and even full marathons, you can help them discover just how strong and amazing they are, and they will want to do more.

We don't stop there! Walking offers so much to so many. While it is perfect for those who are inactive or out of shape, and there are a lot of programs and research on getting people to start walking, once they become regular walkers, programs and researchers tend to forget about them. There are few opportunities for walkers to get additional training to take walking to the next level, and research on the benefits and ways to do this is practically nonexistent. We need to keep this group engaged and challenge them to do more and reap additional benefits. Walking the same route at the same pace over time gets boring—and less effective. You'll learn how to turn ordinary walking into a vigorous workout and to design exciting walking challenges to keep current walkers motivated to meet, even exceed, their goals and expectations. In 8- to 12-week training programs, our walkers have been able to shave an average of 2.5 minutes off their one-mile walk time. With persistence, walkers have even reached speeds of 6.2 miles per hour for 5Ks—without doing formal racewalking.

Walking has a place in the lives of your hard-core clients, too. You'll discover how even marathoners and CrossFit fanatics benefit from walking. Research shows that all the sitting we do throughout the day—even if we work out for an hour a day—can increase risk for heart disease and diabetes. This group, along with everyone else, needs to be educated on the dangers of too much sitting and provided with ways to counteract it—short bouts of walking are the answer.

This simple yet effective workout may also lead to new business alliances. Because walking doesn't cost a lot and most people can do it, employers may be more amenable to having you facilitate a walking program instead of doing other types of workouts. The low risk of injury and accessibility to all fitness levels makes walking programs intriguing prospects for hospitals and doctors. Park and recreation departments are potential partners. Even grocery and drug stores see the potential in walking. Wegmans supermarkets in the United States created the Hit the Trail Passport program to encourage people to get active by exploring area trails. Walgreens supports customers who walk by giving them reward points that can be redeemed for discounts on purchases. Community and religious organizations also provide potential venues for offering walking programs.

The Walking Solution is an exciting addition to your professional toolbox, helping you become a change agent. The important take-home message from this book is that you can use walking as the foundation for an effective and inspirational fitness workout across a broad demographic that traditional fitness programs have not been able to reach.

Our Stories

Just like there are a variety of ways to walk, there are also different ways to coach walkers. In this book, you'll explore a myriad of walking and coaching opportunities to determine what will work best for you. To help you put this information and our recommendations into context, it's important to know who we are and what we do.

Lee Scott

I had been working as a group fitness leader and personal trainer since 1991 when, in the fall of 2000, I was asked to lead an outdoor walking class at the local community center. Despite being skeptical about the ability of walking to give people a challenging workout, I was willing to give it a whirl. For many years, I had experienced low-back pain from years of figure skating and competitive board sailing. As such, it certainly seemed that walking would be a good workout and heal a painful back. That first outdoor power walking class was, without exaggeration, transformational—and not simply because my back issues dissipated. Perhaps it was the fresh air or the lack of mirrors, but the outdoor environment empowered participants in a way that I had never experienced when teaching indoor aerobics classes. In addition, a strong sense of camaraderie was created in that outdoor environment in which people could encourage each other while working out.

From the very beginning, I used interval walking as the basis for all my walking workouts. Participants responded enthusiastically. They felt challenged during the workout and invigorated afterward. It was easy to manage participants who walked at a variety of paces because there was time between the speed intensity intervals to regroup around the coach. Being outdoors was beautiful and inspiring. As a coach, the walking class offered me a greater opportunity to get to know participants in ways the indoor fitness classes did not.

The community center did not offer the walking classes through the winter, but everyone returned enthusiastically for the spring session. In a short time, I realized that participants had missed the walking workouts through the winter months. I also realized that it was possible for people to walk marathons and other races. It now made sense to offer walking classes all year long and to put my coaching energy solidly behind walking as a foundational activity for fitness. I created my walking-centric business, WoW Power Walking, to help people walk for fitness and walk marathons and other races. Since April 2002, I've offered year-round outdoor walking classes, and they are my major source of business revenue.

Classes meet at local parks, coffee shops, or running stores. Because of the minimal capital investment in real estate, business could be started quickly and easily, and changes in walking locations could be easily managed. Business collaborations with cafes and running stores helped my walking business and the local businesses. All classes are posted on my business website, and registration and payment are managed through the site. Classes are offered on a sessional eight-week basis throughout the year, structured around seasonal change. There are options for drop-in or class pass attendance, although I've found that the sessional sign-up results in more consistent class attendance. This has a twofold effect of increasing participant fitness and creating a more robust walking program with high attendance throughout the year. Special events and workshops keep the program fresh and fun. I also give workshops to community walking groups about technique, drill and workout design, and race training plans. Another aspect of my coaching business involves working with clients remotely over the phone and online to help them become walking athletes or coaches.

Michele Stanten

I'm the former fitness director of *Prevention* magazine, where I worked for more than 20 years and where my passion for walking was ignited. When I started at the magazine in 1991, I was teaching group exercise classes at a local health club, and my charge at the magazine was to expand our coverage of fitness beyond walking. While I did that, I came to appreciate how much walking had to offer and how it was often not given the respect it deserved, especially within the fitness industry. Before giving a talk at a local running and walking group, a few women told me that they were "demoted" to the slowest group because they didn't want to run, even though they were walking faster than some of the slow runners. I must have convinced everyone that "walkers are athletes too" (my motto), because I've been invited back to speak for several years since!

During my time at *Prevention,* I wrote and edited many articles and workouts on walking. It gave me the opportunity to review the latest research, speak with the leaders in exercise science, attend conferences where the latest data was presented, and train or walk with top walking experts, coaches, and racewalkers. In fact, I met Lee at one of those conferences, and she became a valuable resource.

A real turning point for me was when I walked the Avon 3-Day Breast Cancer Walk with my mom in 2000. We walked 20 miles a day for three days from Frederick, Maryland, to Washington, D.C. Seeing people young and old, fit and unfit, slim and obese, healthy and unhealthy coming together, supporting each other, and taking on a serious physical challenge was amazing and life changing. It showed me that walking was accessible to all and that it could be an athletic endeavor. I went back to my job at the magazine excited and determined to take walking to the next level.

In 2005, I launched *Prevention*'s marathon walking program and trained thousands of readers to walk marathons across the country, including a group of 100 readers and magazine staff who walked the Marine Corps Marathon in Washington, D.C. The program grew to five or six events a year, including half marathons. During this time, I also wrote my first walking book, *Walk Off Weight,* to help women achieve better results from walking. Unfortunately, a change in management at the magazine ended the marathon program and other walking initiatives in 2010. A year later, I left the magazine to pursue more walking opportunities on my own.

My business model is significantly different from Lee's. About 80 to 90 percent of my revenue comes from content creation: writing books and articles and generating content for online products, programs, and apps, including audio and video formats. All of it is fitness related, with a significant portion of it specific to walking.

In addition, I coach individual walkers and groups, either in person or virtually. Many of the groups I coach are tied to specific events. For example, a local recreation department hired me to do a summer walking program leading groups at different parks throughout the city each week. I also led a training program for a local library's 5K fundraiser. I work with a local half marathon and 5K, both fundraisers for nonprofits, to manage and promote their walking divisions too. As a mom with school-age children and carpooling duties, short-term project-based walking classes fit better with my other responsibilities than running ongoing classes at this time. For me, the goal of the coaching portion of my business is less about generating revenue and more about demonstrating the potential of walking and walkable communities to organizations, businesses, communities, elected officials, and the media.

Joining Forces

After meeting at the American College of Sports Medicine's Walking for Health conference in 2005, we have been collaborating on walking ever since. In the early days, Lee was often a source for Michele's articles and books. When the marathon program at *Prevention* grew, Michele enlisted Lee's services to help coach the groups. Then, we made it our mission to elevate walking in the fitness industry and began presenting at conferences together.

Now we want to share what we've learned with you.

Walking is good for all of us, and so is being outside. It is time for fitness and wellness professionals to combine walking and the outdoors into one powerful fitness program. Its low cost makes it easy to recruit participants and build a business when starting out, and it has the potential for everyone to experience improved mental and physical well-being, social support, and personal contentment. As longtime fitness junkies who have enjoyed just about every fitness trend, Lee and Michele can attest to the benefits and pure joy of walking outside for fitness. As coaches, they have witnessed the transformation of thousands of lives, all because people started walking for fitness. Let's begin the walking journey together as fitness professionals.

ACKNOWLEDGMENTS

This book would not have happened without the persistence and knowledge of my co-author, Michele Stanten, the enthusiasm of our editor, Michelle Maloney, and the support of Human Kinetics. My most heartfelt thanks to all. Over the past 18 years, the walkers I have had the privilege to coach have taught me so much more than books and certifications. I send a special shout-out to those of you who shared your stories for this book. Thank you and keep walking! To my husband, Greg, who puts such great determination into keeping the pace together, thank you for all the miles side by side. To my three sons, Dylan, Devin, Jason—thanks for your patience with so many years of rushed dinners, my weekends away at marathons, and overwhelming walk talk, you are simply the best. And, to my sister, Sue, one of my original walking companions, thank you for always having the best last-minute advice.

—Lee Scott

I've had the pleasure of walking with so many incredible people in my life who have inspired me, taught me, supported me, and challenged me. Thank you all! One of them is Lee Scott, my friend, mentor, and co-author, who's passion for and knowledge of walking is unmatched. It is always an honor to work and walk with you! To our amazing editor, Michelle Maloney, my deepest gratitude for your belief in this project and determination to make it happen. Thank you to the Human Kinetics team for taking it from a dream to a reality. To my husband, Andrew, I cannot express my appreciation enough for your never-ending support in everything I do. To my son, Jacob, your hugs are always a best part of my day and keep me going. To my daughter, Mia, your boundless energy and silliness energize me and make me smile. And to our puppy, Rosie, who makes sure I step away from the computer every day to play and walk.

—Michele Stanten

PART I

WHY WALKING

1

The Power of Walking

Walking is such powerful medicine that in 2015 the surgeon general of the United States not only encouraged Americans to walk more but also asked all levels of government, civic organizations, health care providers, educational institutions, worksites, and even the media to promote walking. This is not surprising when we consider that back in 1978, the director of the National Institute on Aging wrote, "If exercise could be packed into a pill, it would be the single most widely prescribed and beneficial medicine in the nation" [1]. Today, there's even more evidence supporting that statement.

Step It Up! The Surgeon General's Call to Action to Promote Walking and Walkable Communities challenges all sectors of society—including transportation, land use, and community design; parks, recreation, and fitness; education; business and industry; volunteer and nonprofit organizations; health care; media; and public health—to play a role in promoting walking. This aligns with the goal of every health, wellness, and fitness professional: to help people be healthier and happier.

Exercise, including walking, can have a positive effect on 34 chronic diseases or conditions, such as heart disease, diabetes, back pain, and depression. It can help people live longer. Walking an average of 30 minutes a day can lower the risk of heart disease [2], stroke [3], and diabetes [4] by 30 to 40 percent and breast cancer by 20 to 30 percent [5]. A 15-minute walk after every meal improves blood sugar regulation in people with prediabetes [6]. Children with ADHD can benefit. Researchers found that following a walk out in nature, children with ADHD were more focused and better able to complete tasks [7]. Other studies have shown that exercising outdoors improves mood, concentration [8], and even nighttime sleep patterns [9] in adults. Walking is powerful enough to affect our genes. In one study, researchers studied 12,000 people to determine how weight-promoting genes contributed to body weight. Then they looked at the participants' exercise habits. The genetic effect was cut in half in those who walked briskly for an hour a day, meaning they weighed less [10].

The power of walking is not only in the physical and mental benefits it offers but also in its accessibility. People can walk almost anywhere at any time. They can do it alone or in a group. Stepping outside for a walk means that a drive across town to a health club is no longer an obstacle to activity. People can easily walk on their own when they're not with

Walk With a Doc

Case Study

Decades of research have proven the benefits of walking to the point that doctors are now prescribing it to their patients. But even before it became trendy, one doctor took it a step further. In 2005, David Sabgir, a cardiologist in Columbus, Ohio, started inviting his patients to walk with him in the park on Saturdays.

The initiative started out of Dr. Sabgir's frustration in motivating his patients to adopt healthy behaviors. During their appointments, he would spend time talking with them about making healthy lifestyle changes, such as walking and being less sedentary. They would seem committed, but when they returned six months or a year later, nothing had changed. He knew he needed a new approach.

Instead of telling them what to do, Dr. Sabgir decided to show them how to do it. When he invited his patients to the first walk in a park, more than 100 of them showed up. That was the beginning of the Walk with a Doc program. In 14 years, the program has grown to more than 400 chapters around the world, with programs in 47 states in the United States and 21 countries.

Depending upon the program, walks are scheduled weekly, biweekly, or monthly in a local park. They last for an hour and usually have two assistants and a doctor present. During some walks, healthy snacks are provided or blood pressure testing is offered.

The walk kicks off with a three- to five-minute presentation by a doctor on a relevant health topic. The remainder of the time, everyone walks (or rolls if in a stroller or wheelchair) at their own paces. In addition to exercise, it offers an opportunity to build a stronger relationship between the doctors and their patients as they walk and talk. "We ditch our white coats in favor of a ball cap and sneakers," says Dr. Sabgir. "There's laughter, education, and communication on a level that is altering the health care landscape." More than 90 percent of Walk with a Doc participants feel that they are more educated since starting the program. About 80 percent feel more empowered in their interactions with health care providers. And of course, they are getting more exercise!

For more information on Walk with a Doc, go to http://walkwithadoc.org.

you to maximize the benefits they'll get from your training. It also opens a variety of venues where you can offer classes.

Lee runs classes year-round in Toronto, and when the weather is bad, she has done them in empty parking garages. Michele has led classes in empty parking lots. This type of innovative thinking has inspired clients to be creative with how they fit in their workouts. One mother now does walking intervals up and down her driveway when her husband is traveling and she can't leave her sleeping kids home alone. It's also an opportunity to meet people where they are—in their neighborhoods, at parks, in churches. It gets you out into your community and benefits the community as a whole on many levels beyond just health. The more people who are out walking, the safer a community will be, and higher foot traffic in downtown areas tends to boost retail business.

Walking offers an easy way to meet recommended levels of physical activity, yet less than 50 percent of Americans meet these guidelines. Over the past 25 years that we've been a part of the fitness industry, we've seen the introduction of step aerobics, Spinning, elliptical machines, HIIT, boot camp workouts, Pilates, yoga, Tae Bo, Zumba, and dozens of other exercise programs designed to get Americans in shape. Still, the number of Americans who meet the recommended amounts of physical activity hasn't changed. Much of the programming has focused on keeping people who are already exercising engaged by offering bigger, faster, harder workouts. The industry has been engaging the same 15 to 20 percent of the population instead of helping the other 80 percent get the health benefits that physical activity has to offer. As an industry, we haven't made much progress in getting the inactive or minimally active segments of the population moving. Many of these people are intimidated to join a gym, think something like boot camp isn't for them, or may be embarrassed exercising in front of others. Starting with an activity that is accessible and popular, like walking, is a great entry point for this population.

Walking is easy, and everyone knows how to do it. In fact, a recent *Washington Post* article opened with, "Humans are walkers, and we're really good at it" [11]. This builds self-efficacy, the belief in one's self to do something, which has been found to be a key determinant in making behavior changes. Most people believe that they can walk, so they're more likely to stick with a walking program. Achieving early successes—such as walking every day or hitting a step goal—boosts confidence and motivates people to continue. Even when you introduce technique to make walking more effective, the changes are simple, build on each other, and produce fast results. After just one class, walkers can increase speed, giving them another win that will encourage them to keep going.

More Than One Way to Walk

Over 100 million people report that they "walk for exercise," but what does "walk for exercise" mean? Most surveys that track this data don't define it, but if you were to sit in a park and watch people walk, you'd quickly see that there are many ways of walking for exercise. You might see elderly people who need assistance from walkers or canes. But they are still walking for exercise. Others may be strolling while chatting with friends or family. They're getting benefits, too. Some are chugging along like they have someplace to be, and that definitely looks more like exercise. And finally, you might see speedy walkers who are focused, moving with their arms bent, and taking quick steps. On websites, in magazines, on television, and in other types of media, you may see some types of walking referred to as power walking, fitness walking, aerobic walking, or speed walking. There are no standard definitions for the various ways that people walk. To get everyone on the same page, here are our working definitions.

Everyday Walking

Ambling around your house or place of work, trekking to and from your car, shopping, or any other incidental activities that require a little bit of light-intensity walking fall into this category. Researchers refer to this incidental activity as nonexercise activity thermogenesis, or NEAT. While these steps aren't going to improve cardio fitness, recent studies show that they are vital to good health and well-being. Over the past 50 years or so, people are doing less of this type of walking as remote controls, labor-saving devices, and cars have become more prevalent. While you are not going to build classes around this type of walking, it is important to educate your clients on the importance of being active outside of formal exercise sessions. And with the popularity of activity monitors, it's easy to set goals and track progress around this behavior. It has been commonplace to hear recommendations to walk 10,000 steps every day. While counting steps is an easy way to set a goal and track progress, 10,000 steps may not be the right goal for everyone. For more on step counting and using everyday walking in your programs, see the Tracking Daily Steps section in chapter 9.

Leisure Walking

Easy walking or strolling with the arms hanging down at the sides and minimal stopping is considered leisure walking. A leisure walk might involve walking while chatting with a friend, walking the dog, or even walking to do an errand. It is relaxed, and the effort is light enough that a person can sing while walking. A walk at this low-to-moderate level of intensity is great for socializing, relaxing, or getting some fresh air and has similar benefits as everyday walking.

Brisk Walking

When walking becomes more purposeful, it's referred to as brisk, and it starts to count toward meeting the physical activity guideline recommendations for moderate-intensity exercise. Brisk walking is usually what is meant by references to fitness walking. Technique is usually not practiced for this type of walking. Brisk walking can happen at a range of effort levels and a variety of speeds, depending on the individual. This level of intensity induces more labored breathing and an increase in heart rate and may cause people to start sweating. Studies show that if a walker consciously thinks,

"I'm going to walk briskly," they will hit the right stride. If they are looking to become fitter, lose weight, or lower blood glucose or blood pressure, this type of walking improves those health indicators.

Power Walking

We've settled on using the term *power walking* to describe the aerobic or speed walking that you'll learn about in this book. Walking requires that muscle power be activated for each step, in contrast to running. There is no spring action happening through the knee joint during the walk gait, as happens during running. Each step requires active muscle power to go fast and get fit. This type of walking also employs technique to speed up, is usually done at a moderate to vigorous intensity, and will improve cardiorespiratory fitness.

Racewalking

Racewalking, an Olympic sport, is a technical type of walking that is governed by two rules. First, one foot must always be in contact with the ground. Second, the front leg must remain straight from the point of heel contact with the ground until the body passes directly over it. At competitions, racewalkers can be disqualified if they break either of these two rules.

The racewalking technique, which involves more hip rotation, can help increase speed, making it a vigorous activity. Olympic racewalkers may complete a mile in as little as six minutes—that's 10 miles per hour! Although we've both done training in racewalking, we do not coach it because its highly technical nature can be a barrier to accessibility. Still, our four-progression approach to power walking, described in chapter 4, is a good starting point for any client who wants to pursue racewalking.

Interval Walking

Alternating intervals of fast walking with slower walking intervals is the hallmark of a training method once reserved for elite athletes. Recent studies show interval training to be beneficial for all exercisers, and it may even be superior to doing longer, steady-state workouts [12]. By doing short bouts, even as little as 10 seconds, of high-intensity activity, interval walking can be a less intimidating way of getting walkers to push themselves out of their comfort zones and achieve greater benefits. In chapter 5, we go into detail on how to use interval walking to create fun and challenging workouts.

The next time you start to say "just walking" or hear someone saying that, remember that there are more ways to walk than you thought. All offer benefits for a variety of people—and you're the perfect person to share the joy of walking with a wider audience. Chapter 2 gives you a concrete understanding of how the body walks. This information will support the coaching you do to help participants achieve their best walking workout.

References

1. Butler, R.N. 1978. "Exercise, the Neglected Therapy." *The International Journal of Aging and Human Development* 8 (2): 193-95. http://journals.sagepub.com/doi/abs/10.2190/AM1W-RABB-4PJY-P1PK?journalCode=ahdb.
2. Manson, J.E., Hu, F.B., Rich-Edwards, J.W., Colditz, G.A., Stampfer, M.J., Willett, W.C., Speizer, F.E., and Hennekens, C.H. 1999. "A Prospective Study of Walking as Compared With Vigorous Exercise in the Prevention of Coronary Heart Disease in Women." *New England Journal of Medicine* 341 (9): 650-58. www.nejm.org/doi/10.1056/NEJM199908263410904?url_ver=Z39.88-2003&rfr_id=ori:rid:crossref.org&rfr_dat=cr_pub%3dwww.ncbi.nlm.nih.gov.
3. Sattelmair, J.R., Kurth, T., Buring, J.E., and Lee, I.M. 2010. "Physical Activity and Risk of Stroke in Women." *Stroke* 41 (6): 1243-50. www.ncbi.nlm.nih.gov/pmc/articles/PMC2876221.
4. Hu, F.B., Sigal, R.J., and Rich-Edwards, J.W. 1999. "Walking Compared With Vigorous Physical Activity and Risk of Type 2 Diabetes in Women: A Prospective Study." *Journal of the American Medical Association* 282 (15): 1433-39. https://jamanetwork.com/journals/jama/fullarticle/192010.
5. Lee, I.M. 2003. "Physical Activity and Cancer Prevention—Data From Epidemiologic Studies." *Medicine & Science in Sports & Exercise* 35 (11): 1823-27. www.ncbi.nlm.nih.gov/pubmed/14600545.
6. Pahra, D., Sharma, N., Ghai, S., Hajela, A., Bhansali, S., and Bhansali, A. 2017. "Impact of Post-Meal and One-Time Daily Exercise in Patients With Type 2 Diabetes Mellitus: A Randomized Crossover Study." *Diabetology & Metabolic Syndrome* 9: 64-70. www.ncbi.nlm.nih.gov/pmc/articles/PMC5580296.
7. Kuo, F.E. and Taylor, A.F. 2004. "A Potential Natural Treatment for Attention-Deficit/Hyperactivity Disorder: Evidence from a National Study." *American Journal of Public Health* 94 (9): 1580-1586. www.ncbi.nlm.nih.gov/pmc/articles/PMC1448497.
8. Pretty, J., Peacock, J., Sellens, M., Griffin, M. 2005. "The Mental and Physical Health Outcomes of Green Exercise." *International Journal of Environmental Health Research* 15 (5): 319-37. www.ncbi.nlm.nih.gov/pubmed/16416750.
9. Gladwell, V.F., Kuoppa, P., Tarvainen, M.P., and Rogerson, M. 2016. "A Lunchtime Walk in Nature Enhances Restoration of Autonomic Control during Nighttime Sleep: Results From a Preliminary Study." *International Journal of Environmental Research and Public Health* 13: 280-88. https://static1.squarespace.com/static/56e9367020c64742fe062659/t/56fe4cd920c64743836af139/1459506399697/A+Lunchtime+Walk+in+Nature+Enhances+Restoration+of+Autonomic+Control+during+Night.pdf.
10. American Heart Association's Epidemiology and Prevention/Nutrition, Physical Activity and Metabolism 2012 Scientific Sessions. https://www.sciencedaily.com/releases/2012/03/120314142833.htm.
11. Achenbach, J. 2018. "3.6-Million-Year-Old Footprints Suggest Early Human Ancestors Were Excellent Walkers." *Washington Post*, April 23.
12. Masuki, S., Morikawa, M., and Nose, H. 2017. "Interval Walking Training Can Increase Physical Fitness in Middle-Aged and Older People." *Exercise and Sports Science Review* 45 (3): 154–62. https://www.ncbi.nlm.nih.gov/pubmed/28418999.

2

Made for Walking

Each person who walks has a unique pattern of movement called a *gait*. In fact, it is so unique that some criminals have been identified by the way they walk. But gait can change. We walk differently as we age or if we develop injuries. Emotions can be exhibited in the way we walk; for example, we change the way we walk when we are exhilarated compared to when we are feeling down.

Humans are the only mammals that walk and run upright on two legs, an action called *bipedal locomotion*. In *Wanderlust*, author Rebecca Solnit beautifully captures an activity that most of us take for granted.

> *Muscles tense. One leg a pillar, holding the body upright between the earth and sky. The other a pendulum, swinging from behind. Heel touches down. The whole weight of the body rolls forward onto the ball of the foot. The big toe pushes off, and the delicately balanced weight of the body shifts again. The legs reverse position.*

The human body is well designed for walking and has the capacity to go long distances because people tend to walk at the most energy-efficient pace. That means conserving energy for long journeys, which were common for our ancestors. It will be important to consider this tendency as you coach walkers and design walking programs, and we'll discuss it in more detail in the next chapter. But first, let's get acquainted with the inner workings of walking.

As a walking coach, you will find it helpful to have an intimate understanding of human gait from heel strike to toe push-off and from posture to propulsion. The movement is complex despite our cultural tendency to refer to it as "just walking." In this chapter, we'll break down the gait cycle, look at muscle recruitment, and compare walking to running. With a better understanding of the biomechanics of walking, you'll be better equipped to provide a higher level of coaching.

Deconstructing the Gait Cycle

Walking may look and feel like a basic forward motion, but it is quite complex. While the main action of walking occurs in the sagittal plane (see Anatomical Planes of Motion section), there is movement across

Anatomical Planes of Motion

Anatomical planes are imaginary lines that divide the human body into sections (figure 2.1). The planes are common in science and are used to locate and define body parts, structures, and anatomical movement. The three primary planes follow.

- *Frontal (or coronal)*—divides body into anterior (front) and posterior (back) portions
- *Sagittal*—divides body into right and left sides
- *Transverse*—divides body into top and bottom

There are also movements within each of these planes.

- Frontal (or coronal) plane movement is lateral; for example, shuffling side to side occurs in the frontal (or coronal) plane.
- Sagittal plane movement is forward or back, like walking or running.
- Transverse plane movement is rotational; an example of this is taking dishes out of the dishwasher and twisting the upper body to put them on the counter.

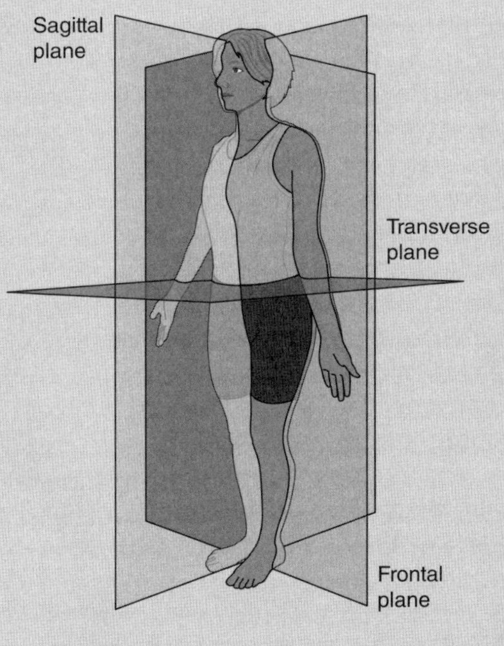

FIGURE 2.1 How the planes divide the body.

all planes happening within the body during the gait cycle—much of it unnoticeable to the average observer. Hips abduct and adduct, moving in the frontal (or coronal) plane, while the pelvis, hips, knees, and even feet rotate in the transverse plane. The gait cycle consists of all events that occur from one footstep to the next. When walking, at least one foot is always on the ground.

Phases of the Gait Cycle

There are two primary phases of the gait cycle: the stance phase and the swing phase. The stance phase is when one or both feet are in contact with the ground. The swing phase is when one foot is in the air. The stance phase accounts for about 60 percent of the cycle, while the swing phase occurs during the remaining 40 percent. The stance phase can be further broken down into single support, when only one foot is on the ground, and double support, when both feet are on the ground.

Double Support Stance Phase

The double support stance phase in the gait cycle is when one foot is landing out in front. Both feet are on the ground, with the front foot landing on the heel and the back foot on the ball of the foot and toes. The hip of the front leg is flexed, the knee extended, and the ankle dorsiflexed (toes pulled toward the shin). The hip of the back leg is extended, the knee slightly flexed, and the ankle plantar flexed (pointing). A snapshot at this point of walking would reveal the lower extremities forming a triangle with the ground and the upper body, including the center of mass (COM) right above in the middle, creating the top point (figure 2.2).

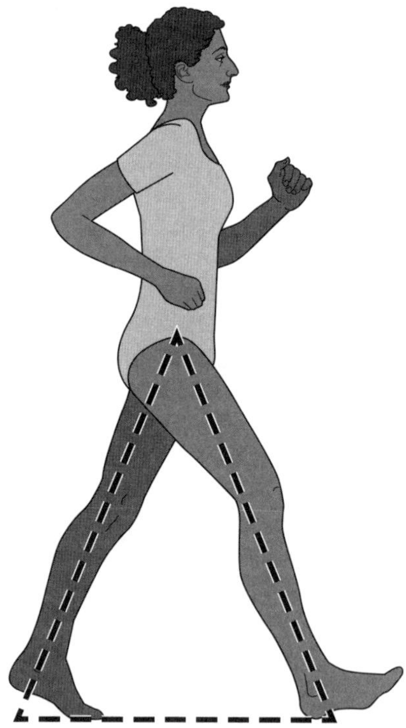

FIGURE 2.2 Double stance triangle. In this position, the legs look like they form a triangle with the ground.

The COM of the body is the point at which opposite sides would be equal in mass if the body were cut in half on any plane (see previous Anatomical Planes of Motion section). If the body were suspended from that point, it would be in perfect balance. The COM is usually about an inch behind the navel but shifts slightly as body positions change. The movement of the COM is a key area of study in gait analysis. For coaching purposes, it's important to understand the basic effects of COM on walking. Before taking a step, when the legs are together, the COM is easily supported by both legs. When in double support stance, neither leg is under the body, so the COM has no direct support, and the weight is pressing straight down toward the ground. With the legs at angles to the torso, it's harder to support the COM. We'll discuss this concept further in chapter 3, as it relates to walking speed.

The double support stance occurs twice during a gait cycle: at the beginning and the end with the legs in opposite positions. At these brief points, body weight is about evenly supported between both legs. While the stance phase accounts for 60 percent of the gait cycle, the double support part of it is very short. In a split second (even faster as speed increases) the heel of the front foot lands, and as the body rolls forward onto the front foot, the back foot pushes off, ending the double support stance phase.

Swing Phase

When the back foot peels off the ground, the swing phase begins as body weight shifts to the front leg as the back leg moves forward. To facilitate the swing, the ankle of the back leg dorsiflexes (pulling toes toward the shin), the knee flexes, and the hip on that side lifts a bit. As the leg swings forward, it catches up to the torso, and together the torso and leg come up onto the supporting leg, and then the back leg becomes the front leg swinging forward. The hip flexes and the knee extends, preparing for landing, and the opposite leg will enter the swing phase.

Single Support Stance Phase

This phase happens simultaneously with the swing phase. While one leg is in the swing phase, the other is in the single support stance phase. The single support phrase begins after the heel strike as the body moves forward onto the front foot, accepting all the body weight onto that leg to allow the back foot to come off the ground. While it is not noticeable to the average person, the body actually slows down during this period of the gait cycle. As the body, including the COM, moves on top of the front leg, it becomes easier to support body weight compared to when the leg is out in front. (You'll see in Take Short Steps in chapter 4 how this affects walking speed.) When the body is directly above the supporting leg and the swinging leg is directly below the body, this position is called *midstance*. From there, the body accelerates as it moves in front of the support leg, continuing the single support stance phase until the heel of the opposite leg lands on the ground for the double support stance phase. Then the single support stance phase will begin for the opposite leg (figure 2.3).

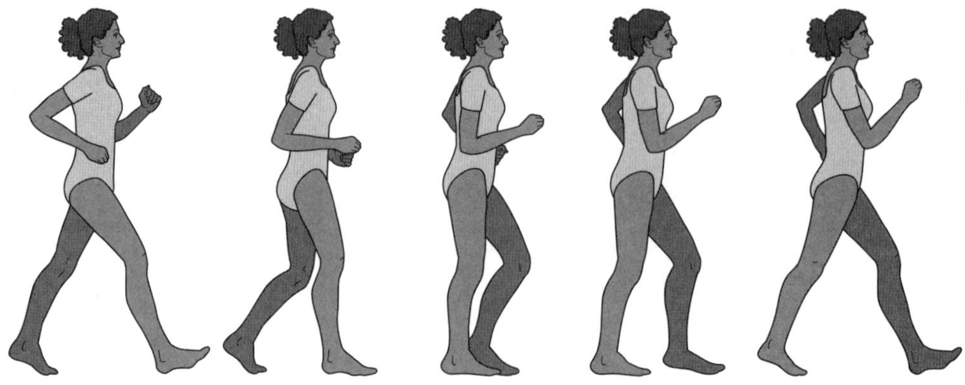

FIGURE 2.3 An illustrated overview of the gait cycle: (a) double stance; (b) single stance (right leg), swing phase (left leg); (c) midstance; (d) single stance (right leg), swing phase (left leg); (e) double stance

Walking Descriptions

The action of walking has been described in a variety of ways, including an inverted pendulum, pole vaulting, and a series of forward falls. Understanding these models will help you coach your walkers to faster, smoother strides.

Inverted Pendulum

A pendulum is a weight hung from a fixed point that swings freely. When thinking about pendulums and walking, it is common to think of the arms and legs as swinging like pendulums. We even use this analogy in coaching, for example, telling walkers that shorter pendulums move faster, so bending the arms will enable them to swing faster. But for the walking model, the pendulum flips. The fixed point is the supporting leg, and the COM is the weight moving forward, but in this case, the fixed point of the pendulum moves with every step. Looking at this model of walking (figure 2.4), you see how the body has to work after the heel strikes the ground to bring the COM over the top of the supporting leg. As the supporting leg goes behind, the COM comes down. So, within walking, there is vertical movement; however, for an efficient stride, other parts of the body, like the pelvis and shoulders, adjust, making the up-and-down motion barely noticeable. (Later in this chapter and in chapter 4, you'll learn what to do when it is noticeable, so you can help people walk more efficiently.) A pendulum continues to swing by converting the kinetic energy of motion into gravitational potential energy and back again. Walking is an exchange of kinetic and potential energy: kinetic energy as the foot lands and the body weight comes up onto the front leg, kind of like pole vaulting body weight over the leg. Then potential energy takes over as the body comes forward in front of the supporting leg, similar to falling and taking advantage of gravity. And so it continues with each step.

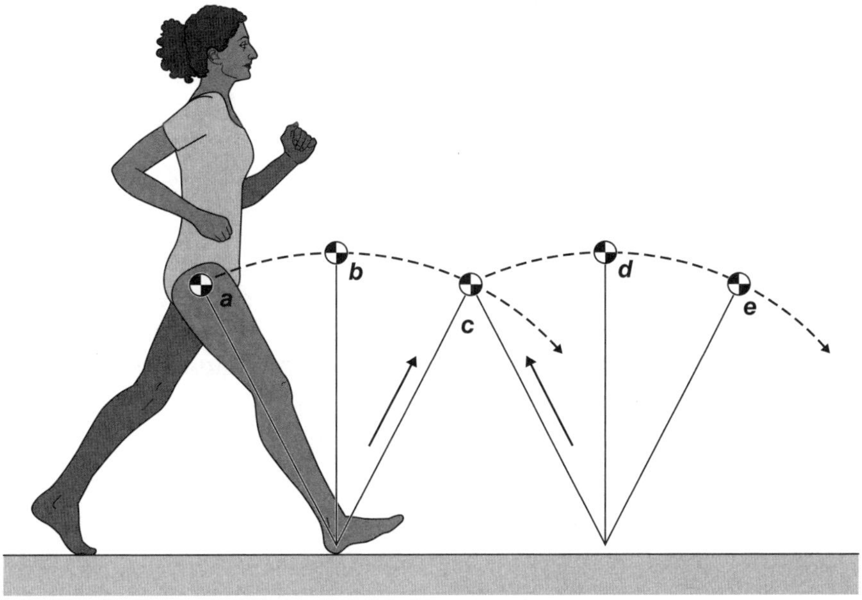

FIGURE 2.4 The inverted pendulum model of walking shows how the body has to work to bring the COM up and over the supporting leg: (a) double stance, (b) midstance, (c) double stance, (d) midstance, (e) double stance

Pole Vaulting

The analogy of walking to pole vaulting helps illustrate the acceleration and deceleration of the body during walking. As the vaulter plants the pole, the action slows as they lift off the ground and fly up toward the bar. It can almost seem as if it's happening in slow motion, and at the top of the movement, it appears that the action stops briefly before it speeds up again as the vaulter falls. Think of the pole vaulter as the body's COM. The heel strike is the pole planting, and the body decelerates as the COM comes up over the supporting leg. Then it accelerates as it falls forward until the heel lands on the ground, slowing things down again.

Falling Forward

Walking has been described as a series of falls in a forward direction. The idea of falling being part of walking was hinted at in the pole-vaulting model. From midstance, where the body is supported on one leg as the other leg just passes underneath, it falls forward. The swinging leg steps out in front and breaks the fall (double support stance). From midstance to double support, the body is falling forward. The fall is the acceleration stage of walking, but when the foot lands, it stops the acceleration, acting almost like a brake. Then comes the deceleration stage. This stage is like climbing, so it's not surprising that speed decreases slightly. The COM moves over the support leg before it falls again. All these changes in speed and up-and-down motion are subtle and usually imperceptible, but they can make a difference in performance. This model has important implications as we discuss increasing speed in chapter 3.

Muscle Actions

Along with kinetic and potential energy, muscles play a large role in powering the walking stride. By understanding which muscles are working when, you'll be better able to help your clients activate the right muscles at the right times. Training these key walking muscles outside of walking workouts will produce more power when walking.

Let's look at the muscle actions as they happen through the gait cycle, following just one leg all the way through.

Stance Phase

As the heel strikes the ground, the gluteus maximus (buttocks) and hamstrings (back of thigh) work to decelerate the body, while some quadriceps (front of thigh) activity kicks in to stabilize the knee on impact. At the same time, the anterior tibialis (shin) is firing to keep the toes up as the heel contacts the ground. Then it begins a lengthening contraction, gradually lowering the rest of the foot to the ground to prevent it from slapping down. As body weight comes onto the front foot, and you move into midstance, the gluteus medius (hip) contracts isometrically to stabilize the pelvis. As the foot moves behind your body, the glutes and hamstrings work to extend the hip. The calf muscles—the gastrocnemius and soleus—are also activated with a final powerful contraction as the foot pushes off the ground behind you and the body propels forward.

Swing Phase

To swing the back leg forward, the iliopsoas (hip) and hamstring (back of thigh) contract to bend the hip and knee, respectively, and lift the leg off the ground. Then, the anterior tibialis (shin) kicks in to dorsiflex the foot so it doesn't touch the ground as the leg swings forward. Finally, the quadriceps (front of thigh) extend the leg in preparation for landing.

Walking Versus Running

We're not looking to create a competition or start a debate when we compare walking to running. The goal is to educate about the differences between walking and running because they are often lumped together. Walking is not simply slow running. We've trained many clients who can zip past recreational joggers, and we (and our clients) have completed half and full marathons ahead of many runners. The difference between the two is not about speed.

The most basic and obvious difference is that at any speed, a walker will always have one foot on the ground. Runners, however, are airborne without either foot on the ground during a significant portion of each stride, especially as they run faster. Running is a high-impact activity, resulting in impact forces equal to anywhere from two to four times body weight. Walking is low impact, with impact forces of usually one to two times body weight. As a result, runners are more likely than walkers to

Wayfinding

Case Study

In March of 2014, Lee and Michele were meeting in Atlanta's Hartsfield-Jackson International Airport while on their way to a conference. Michele arrived first and headed toward the international terminal, where Lee would be arriving. When she found the airport shuttle, Michele asked an airport attendant if it was possible to walk to the international terminal instead. "You can, but it's really far. I don't think you want to do that," was the response she got. Michele walked anyway, and it took less than 20 minutes.

Fast forward six months, when the Centers for Disease Control and Prevention launched their Walk to Fly study at Atlanta's airport. The study involved posting four strategically located signs that encouraged walking by letting passengers know that it was only a five-minute walk between concourses. After the signs were posted, 11 to 17 percent more people per day walked between concourses compared to when there was no signage [2].

The signs at Atlanta airport are a pedestrian wayfinding system, a navigational system that helps people orient to where they are and navigate from place to place. Even before pedestrian wayfinding found itself in airports, it was used in cities.

Traditionally, most signage in cities is directed at motorists. But in recent years, cities have become more interested in encouraging walking for a variety of reasons. In addition to improving health, increased pedestrian traffic can improve the economy, make areas safer, reduce traffic congestion, and decrease pollution. To do that, cities like Charlotte, North Carolina; Philadelphia, Pennsylvania; and New York City have invested in pedestrian wayfinding systems. These systems communicate that walking to many destinations is possible and encourage residents and visitors to walk more and drive less. Since people have a better understanding of time than mileage, the signs focus on the time it will take to walk to a specific location. While research on wayfinding to encourage walking is limited, preliminary findings suggest it can have a positive effect.

Pedestrian wayfinding systems can also be used in settings such as hospitals, universities, corporate campuses, industrial parks, and community parks.

For more information, go to http://americawalks.org/create-a-pedestrian-wayfinding-system.

sustain an injury, based on numerous studies. According to the Aerobics Center Longitudinal Study that included nearly 4,000 walkers and runners, walkers reported 25 percent fewer injuries than runners [1]. For both activities, impact increases with speed. However proper training, such as appropriate foot landing, appears to minimize impact in elite runners and racewalkers, who experience less impact forces compared to recreational runners and racewalkers.

Another key difference between walking and running is the energy produced by each activity. Walking is an exchange of kinetic energy from motion and gravitational potential energy. Running is an exchange of kinetic energy and elastic potential energy. Elastic energy is like a spring. As a runner lands on the ground, elastic energy is stored in tendons and muscles and enables the runner to again spring off the ground. Think of it like a ball bouncing back up off the ground. Walking is a little more like tossing a ball. Gravitational potential energy kicks in as the ball is falling. It would be reasonable to say that repetitively bouncing a ball is easier than tossing one. However, most people would say that running is harder than walking. While that's true at a preferred walking speed, effort changes at faster speeds, and some of that relates to the energy produced. That's why as you try to walk faster, you get to a point in which it would feel easier to run and take advantage of the elastic energy. We'll explore this concept more in chapter 3.

Common Gait Deviations

As you begin to coach walkers, you will probably see deviations from typical gait patterns. Many things can affect a person's gait, from age and body size to injuries and style of shoes. As a walking coach, you're not expected to do gait analysis on your clients. In fact, you should refrain from doing it unless you have training. However, common deviations can be corrected or at least minimized as you teach people good posture and techniques. You can watch for other atypical gait patterns, offer basic advice when appropriate, and know when to refer to health care professionals. Sometimes gait problems can have a neurological cause such as Parkinson's disease, so it's always a good idea to encourage clients to see their doctors.

You'll learn how to coach good walking posture and techniques to counteract some of these deviations in chapter 4.

Rounded Upper Body and Looking Down

You've seen that hunched-over posture that many people assume when they're in front of their computers, on their phones, or sitting behind the wheel in their cars. Sadly, many people bring that poor posture to walking.

Spending too much time in this posture can cause weak back muscles and tight chest muscles. The strength training programs in chapter 7 are specially designed to address this issue. Other people assume this position because they are worried about tripping and falling. (You'll find advice on how to coach walking technique to address this concern in chapter 4.) It's also a common response to walking in cold, windy weather, so dressing appropriately can improve posture. When people straighten up, they look and feel better, and walking becomes easier. In some cases, especially in older adults, the rounded posture could be the result of a spinal disorder called kyphosis, which is an exaggerated curvature of the thoracic (upper back) spine. Osteoporosis, arthritis, and poor posture are common contributors to kyphosis. You should encourage anyone with this condition to see a doctor to treat the underlying cause, which will make walking easier.

Bending at the Waist

When people start to walk for exercise, they tend to be enthusiastic and ready to go, go, go. They want to get moving and sometimes end up bending at the waist and leading with their heads out in front of their bodies. This misaligned posture puts tremendous stress on the low back, especially when walking longer distances. Simply making people aware of what they are doing, showing them proper posture, and reminding them to stand tall will usually correct the problem.

Bouncing

Despite the rise and fall of the COM discussed previously, walking should not appear to be an up-and-down motion. Bouncing when walking is usually caused by an improper push-off or excessive striding. Instead of pushing off forward to propel the body in that direction, the walker will push off with upward momentum. Or they are taking too long of a stride. A walker who bounces often walks on their toes. Training in proper push-off and foot motion (chapter 4) can help.

Arm Swing

Once you start watching people walk, you may be amazed to see the various ways that people move their arms while walking—punching forward, winging their elbows out to the sides, swinging their arms across their bodies, flailing arms, and much more. All this upper-body movement can affect gait. At the very least, it's not efficient and slows pace. Teaching proper arm swing (Progression 1 section of chapter 4) is usually effective in correcting these less-efficient movements.

More Challenging Gait Deviations

These patterns tend to be seen less often and aren't as easily adjusted with basic training. In some cases, you should recommend that clients see a doctor.

Foot Slapping

A loud, slapping landing signals that a walker is landing flat-footed instead of striking the ground first with the heel and then rolling onto the midfoot, ball of the foot, and finally the toes. Simply making someone aware of the sound their feet are making and instructing them in the proper foot roll will correct the problem. Another cause may be related to the shoes they are wearing. A stiff shoe will make it more difficult to roll from heel to toes, causing the foot to hit the ground more quickly, even if they are landing on their heel. This issue may also be caused by weak ankle dorsiflexors, such as the anterior tibialis (shin). For exercises to strengthen this area, see shin area exercises in chapter 7. If the problem persists, encourage your client to see a doctor. Sometimes it may be due to a neurological issue.

Foot Scuffing

This occurs when the foot of the swinging leg skims the ground as it is coming forward. This can happen if the supporting leg is bent instead of being fully extended. Similar to foot slapping, it may also be caused by weak ankle dorsiflexors such as the anterior tibialis. Another cause could be weak core muscles that are allowing the hip to drop. If you only notice the problem toward the end of a session, fatigue may be a contributor. If the problem persists, recommend that your client consult with a health professional.

Upper-Body Sway

If you notice the upper body swaying, check foot position. Side-to-side movement of the upper body is often the result of walking with the feet spread too far apart in the frontal plane. Feet should be positioned under the pelvis, as parallel as possible, and close together, no more than four inches apart. A wide foot position slows you down, while a narrower one allows you to go faster by reducing sideways motion of the upper body and directing your energy forward, the direction you want to be going.

An upper-body sway while walking may also result from weak hip abductor muscles, like the gluteus medius, gluteus minimus, and tensor fasciae latae. These muscles are responsible for keeping the pelvis level, especially during the single support stance phase. When they're not working properly, the pelvis on the opposite side of the weakness will drop. To compensate, the upper body will lean toward the weak side to keep the pelvis level. This gait pattern is called *Trendelenburg gait* and is often seen in older adults. In a 2016 study [3] published in the journal *Human Movement Science*, researchers studied the effects of Trendelenburg gait at the knee. When 15 healthy individuals mimicked the Trendelenburg gait, inward movement of the knee increased by up to 25 percent. This results in increased load at the knee, which over time may result in increased wear and tear of the cartilage in the joint, pain, and even an increased risk of osteoarthritis. If you suspect this in any of your clients, encourage them to see a doctor, such as a physiatrist (physical medicine and rehab doctor; see What Is a Physiatrist? section in chapter 12).

Now that you have a better understanding of the mechanics of walking, start to watch people walk. Identify the stages of the gait cycle, and notice variations in the ways people walk. Notice how gait changes as people go faster. The more you observe, the more your coaching skills will be enhanced, reinforcing what you are learning and building knowledge that you'll be able to share with your clients. Next, part II contains two chapters that address how to intentionally intensify the walking pace and how to coach proper technique to make that pace more easily achievable.

References

1. Colbert, L.H., Hootman, J.M., and Macera, C.A. 2000. "Physical Activity-Related Injuries in Walkers and Runners in the Aerobics Center Longitudinal Study." *Clinical Journal of Sports Medicine* 10 (4):259-63. www.ncbi.nlm.nih.gov/pubmed/11086751.
2. Fulton, J.E., Frederick, G.M., Paul, P., Omura, J.D., Carlson, S.A., and Dorn, J.M. 2017. "Increasing Walking in the Hartsfield-Jackson Atlanta International Airport: The Walk to Fly Study." *American Journal of Public Health* 107 (7): 1143-49. www.ncbi.nlm.nih.gov/pubmed/28520493.
3. Dunphy, C., Casey, S., Lomond, A., and Rutherford, D. 2016. "Contralateral Pelvic Drop During Gait Increases Knee Adduction Movements of Asymptomatic Individuals." *Human Movement Science* 49: 27-35. www.sciencedirect.com/science/article/abs/pii/S0167945716300756.

PART II

THE NEW WAY TO WALK

3

Intensify the Pace

Walking is often pigeonholed as a low- to moderate-intensity workout. For example, in the 2018 Physical Activity Council's Annual Study Tracking Sports, Fitness, and Recreation Participation in the US, "walking for fitness" is categorized as a low calorie-burning activity, along with stretching, bowling, and snowmobiling [1]. In the 2008 Physical Activity Guidelines issued by the US Department of Health and Human Services, racewalking was classified as vigorous activity. All other types of walking found in the Guidelines are listed as moderate intensity [2].

Walking isn't usually thought of as a vigorous activity because most people don't walk vigorously. The human body was designed for low-intensity, long-distance walking. Humans naturally select an energy-efficient walking pace—meaning fewer calories are burned. Studies show that this natural pace is about 2.8 to 3.1 miles per hour (or about 21 to 19 minutes per mile). Even regular walkers doing it for exercise tend to self-select a pace of about 3.5 miles per hour (17 min per mile). Many walkers don't realize that they can get faster, or they don't know how to speed up without starting to run. This is where you as a walking coach can be a valued asset. Before we discuss the details for helping walkers get faster, let's look at the potential walking has to be a vigorous activity and why it's worth the extra effort to speed up.

Why Walk Faster?

You probably know walkers who've been walking for years at the same distance and pace. Walking is similar to other types of exercise in that the body becomes accustomed to a particular activity and plateaus if things are not changed up to increase the challenge. The same is true of walking. One of the easiest and most time-efficient ways to change a walking program is to speed up. The benefits a walker receives from getting faster are not only physical, such as reducing risk of disease, burning more calories, and maybe even losing more weight, but also psychological, such as a boost in confidence and a sense of accomplishment from challenging themselves and seeing progress.

It Saves Time

In general, people get all the wonderful benefits of exercise in less time by walking faster. Considering that "I don't have time" is one of the most common excuses for not exercising, a walking plan that delivers results with shorter workouts can be appealing to a broad range of clients and may be a useful marketing angle for you. The Physical Activity Guidelines even recommend substituting vigorous activity for moderate-intensity activity as a "time-efficient way to achieve greater fitness and health goals" [3].

It Enhances Benefits

Along with being more time-efficient, picking up the pace can amplify the benefits of walking.

Vigorous activity most clearly has an advantage over moderate-intensity activity in terms of cardiorespiratory fitness as measured by $\dot{V}O_2max$. The harder the exercise, the stronger the heart gets. A classic study from the Cooper Institute for Aerobics Research published in *The Journal of the American Medical Association* in 1991 [4] clearly shows the benefit of walking faster. Researchers had 102 sedentary women, ages 20 to 40, walk 3 miles 5 days a week for 24 weeks. One group strolled at 3 miles per hour (20 min per mile), another walked briskly at 4 miles per hour (15 min per mile), a third group built up to walking 5 miles per hour (12 min per mile), and one group did not exercise. The results: Brisk walkers improved their $\dot{V}O_2max$ more than twice as much as the strollers while the fast walkers' gains were four times as much. The faster walkers also improved body composition, losing fat and gaining muscle, even though they were a healthy weight to start.

And remember the preference we mentioned about shorter workouts? According to reports from the walking coach who worked on the study, they had a harder time keeping the strollers in the study because their workouts took longer. The strollers had to go for an hour to complete the three miles while the brisk walkers were done in 45 minutes, and the fast walkers wrapped up their workouts in 36 minutes. For many people, hearing that they can cut their workout time almost in half is all they need to motivate them to push themselves to walk faster.

Cardiorespiratory fitness isn't the only heart benefit that fast walking has to offer. In the Women's Health Initiative observational study, a prospective study that followed nearly 75,000 women ages 50 to 79 for up to six years, researchers tracked exercise habits to see their effects on the prevention of cardiovascular disease. Women who walked 2.5 hours a week reduced the risk of having a cardiovascular event like a heart attack by about 30 percent. When they looked more closely, though, they found greater protection at faster speeds. Women who strolled between 2 and 3 miles per hour (30 to 20 min per mile) reduced their risk by 14 percent. Brisk walkers going 3 to 4 miles per hour (20 to 15 min per mile), cut the

$\dot{V}O_2$max As a Measure of Fitness

Oxygen uptake is commonly known as maximal oxygen uptake or $\dot{V}O_2$max. This measurement is considered the most relevant measurement of cardiorespiratory fitness because it represents the transportation and utilization of oxygen in the body during maximal (max) exercise as described as volume (V) of oxygen (O_2) used: hence, $\dot{V}O_2$max. There are several ways to determine $\dot{V}O_2$max, and it is most accurately measured in laboratory settings with specialized equipment. Still, you may want to determine $\dot{V}O_2$max outside of a laboratory fitness test. You can do so by first determining the client's resting heart rate. It can be measured with a heart rate monitor or by taking a pulse at the wrist or carotid artery at the neck when they are at rest. Next, determine your client's theoretical maximal heart rate by subtracting their age from 220. Then, insert these values into the $\dot{V}O_2$max equation, which is $\dot{V}O_2\text{max} = 15 \times (\text{HRmax/HRrest})$.

It may be useful to have clients know their resting heart rates even if you do not calculate their $\dot{V}O_2$max. Resting heart rate is a marker of fitness, and it typically decreases as fitness improves. A once-a-week check on resting heart rate can be a good way to track fitness improvement with walk training—a great way for people to have tangible evidence that exercise is making a difference!

risk by 24 percent. Speedy walkers clocking in at more than 4 miles per hour (15 min per mile) tripled their protection. They lowered their risk by 42 percent [5]. Some of the protection may come from the positive effects on cholesterol. In a six-month study published in the *Archives of Internal Medicine*, sedentary individuals who followed a high-intensity walking program saw greater improvements in their HDL (good) cholesterol than those who did a moderate-intensity walking program [6].

Even for people with hypertension and heart disease, a faster walking pace offers protection. When researchers analyzed the walking speeds of more than 1,000 hypertensive patients, they found that the faster walkers (averaging 3.2 mph) spent less time in the hospital than intermediate- (averaging 2.4 mph) or slow-paced (averaging 1.6 mph) walkers, according to the results of a three-year study presented at the 2018 European Society of Cardiology conference [7]. More than half of the slow walkers had at least one hospitalization compared to less than one-third of the faster walkers. The slow group also spent more than four times as many total days in the hospital as the fast group (4,186 versus 990), and their average length of stay was more than three times as long (23 versus 9 days).

The faster the walking speed, the greater the impact forces on the body. Although the level of impact remains much lower than running, fast walking appears to have a more beneficial effect on bones than slower speeds. Belgian researchers analyzed the forces of a variety of types of exercise on the femoral neck (the top of the thigh bone), which is a common site for osteoporosis-related fractures. As expected, jumping and running had the greatest potential for improving bone strength. The 2018 study, published in the journal *PLOS One*, showed that faster walking speeds are more likely than slower ones or even resistance exercises targeting this area to improve bone density [8]. That may be one of the reasons that the Nurses' Health Study published in the *Journal of the American Medical Association*, an analysis of more than 61,000 women ages 40 to 77, found that women who walked at a brisk to very brisk pace had a 65 percent lower risk of having a hip fracture than sedentary women, compared to 49 percent for women walking at an easy pace [9].

Increasing pace improves the benefits to the brain that already begin with even moderate activity levels. At higher workout intensities, serotonin—a neurotransmitter that improves mood—is manufactured more readily [10]. Additionally, a protein called Brain Derived Neurotrophic Factor (BDNF) is made in greater amounts to help build new neurons [11]. We feel happier, and we are smarter.

Faster walkers may even live longer. In a 2014 University of Pennsylvania study, researchers tracked about 5,000 older adults for an average of 13.5 years and found that those who walked at speeds faster than 100 steps per minute had a 21 percent reduction in all-cause mortality during the study. The reduction in risk got greater as they got faster. For each increase of 10 steps per minute, an additional 4 percent reduction was seen [12].

Burn Calories Like a Runner

According to the *Compendium of Physical Activities* [13], walking and running at 5 miles per hour burns a similar number of calories per minute. Other research shows that walking at faster speeds bumps up calorie burn at a greater rate than running at a similar pace. When healthy women increased their walking speed from 5 to 5.5 miles per hour, they torched 21 percent more calories while the same change in running speed provided a mere 7 percent boost, according to a Washington University School of Medicine study published in the *Journal of Sports Medicine and Physical Fitness* [14]. Surprisingly, when they kicked it up to 6 miles per hour, there was no related increase in calorie burn for runners, but walkers got another 16 percent boost, burning an average of 10 calories per minute versus 7.5 calories per minute for running. Some of the differences in calorie burn are likely attributed to the different types of energy that each activity uses. Running uses elastic potential energy, which is like having springs on the feet. When a runner lands, the elastic energy helps to propel them forward, like a bouncing ball. Walking has less elastic potential energy available, which means more muscle power is required to gain speed. This is why at faster speeds it feels easier to run.

Even if these higher speeds can't be reached, training to crank it up over 4 miles per hour (15 min per mile) offers a bigger calorie burn boost. According to a 2006 study in the *British Journal of Sports Medicine* [15], walkers in their 50s burned 32 percent more calories when they adjusted their speed from 4.1 to 4.6 miles per hour (15 to 13 min per mile) compared with only a 25 percent boost from 3.6 to 4.1 miles per hour (17 to 15 min per mile). In each case, walking only a half mile per hour faster results in an exponentially greater calorie burn. As walking speed increases, walking becomes a less efficient mode of locomotion, meaning it's harder to do. At these speeds, running becomes the easier activity biomechanically (not in terms of the impact on joints or the challenge to the cardiorespiratory system), as discussed in the previous chapter. The increase in calorie burn with faster speeds may be helpful for walkers whose goals involve weight loss.

It Feels Amazing

No, not the actual act of pushing to go faster (although some do enjoy the challenge) but the feeling of accomplishment. When walkers see that hard work is paying off by logging a faster one-mile finish time, completing a particular route quicker than ever before, counting more steps during a fast interval (Counting Steps section of chapter 5), or setting a personal best at a 10K, half marathon, or other race, they get a confidence boost that often propels them to keep it up. It can also make walking more fun and solidifies their commitment to it.

Is It Really Possible to Walk That Fast?

We've trained walkers up to speeds of 6.3 miles per hour (9.5 min per mile) without coaching formal racewalking (Olympic racewalkers can reach speeds of 10 miles per hour, a 6-min-per-mile pace). In a typical 8- to 12-week training program, walkers on average cut their one-mile walk time by 2.5 minutes. Slower walkers, who took 18 or more minutes to walk a mile initially, averaged a 3-minute reduction in their time. And even fast walkers, who clocked under 15 minutes for the mile before training, got speedier, averaging nearly a 1.5-minute reduction.

In the Cooper Institute for Aerobics Research study [16], sedentary women ages 20 to 40 trained and were able to maintain a pace of 5 miles per hour (12 min per mile) for three miles. While it was challenging, they were no more likely to get injured than the slower walkers, nor were they more likely to drop out of the program. The women in the Washington University School of Medicine study previously mentioned were younger with an average age of 27, but they were able to reach even higher speeds and maintain them for five minutes without the formal training offered in the Cooper study. All the women were able to walk at 5 miles per hour (12 min per mile), and half of them were able to hit 6.5 miles per hour (9.25 min per mile) for five minutes.

Even if your clients (or you) cannot hit these higher speeds, there are benefits to be had from any increase.

How Exercise Should Feel

You are responsible for pushing walkers out of their comfort zone. They may not feel comfortable with the effort. This is normal. Still, some symptoms aren't normal and should not be ignored. Here are guidelines on how exercise should feel, what's abnormal, and what to do if anyone experiences any of these symptoms. Educate your walkers on the differences.

There may be situations where you should suggest a participant be cleared by a doctor. These include, but are not restricted to, chronic medical conditions such as diabetes, high blood pressure, or arthritis or factors that put them at a higher risk, such as smoking or being overweight by more than 20 pounds.

NORMAL	ABNORMAL	What to do
Heart pumping rhythmically harder and faster	Chest pain, pressure, or tightness; skipped heartbeats or palpitations	Stop immediately and call 911.
Breathing faster and harder	Shortness of breath, can't catch your breath upon easing up	Stop immediately. If shortness of breath persists after stopping, call 911. If it eases, but the occurrence was unusual or happens again, call your doctor.
Muscle soreness or burning	Sharp, shooting pain or pain in a joint	Stop, rest, and ice the area. If pain persists, see a doctor.
General fatigue	Lightheaded or dizziness	Stop immediately. If lightheadedness or dizziness persists after stopping, transport to a safe location and call your doctor.

Finding Vigorous

There are a variety of ways to evaluate intensity to help you and your clients determine if they are hitting the mark.

One way of defining intensity is to use metabolic equivalents, or METs. This unit of measurement describes the energy expenditure of specific activities. One MET is the rate of energy expended at rest. So, a 5.0-MET activity expends five times the amount of energy used by the body at rest. Moderate-intensity activities are defined as those that are 3.0 to 5.9 METS.

Vigorous activities are those with MET values of 6.0 or higher. Those under 3.0 METs would be light or low intensity [17].

The *Compendium of Physical Activities* is a standardized listing of MET values for hundreds of activities, ranging from playing instruments and doing home repairs to conditioning exercises and sports, and all the values are based on scientific research. The compendium was developed to help standardize physical activity intensity in epidemiological research. Based on the latest update of the compendium in 2011, walking at 4.5 miles per hour on level ground is 7 METs—clearly a vigorous activity. A 3.0-miles-per-hour pace is 3.5 METs. A 3.5-miles-per-hour pace is 4.3 METs, and a 4.0-miles-per-hour pace is 5.0 METs—all within the moderate-intensity level. Because all these values are supported by published research, they're very reliable data to show that walking can be a vigorous form of exercise.

A 2019 study, published in the *International Journal of Behavioral Nutrition and Physical Activity*, quantified thresholds of moderate intensity (3 METs) and vigorous intensity (6 METs) walking based on step cadence [18]. After testing 76 healthy adults between the ages of 21 and 40, researchers from the University of Massachusetts, Amherst, found that moderate intensity begins at 100 steps per minute and vigorous intensity at 130 steps per minute.

Intensity is also relative to a person's fitness level. A very fit person may be working at a moderate intensity when doing a 6.0-MET activity, while an unfit person may be exercising vigorously when doing a 4.0-MET activity. A University of Virginia study [19] that looked at the effects of high- and low-intensity exercise in a group of overweight middle-aged women is a good example of the relativity of intensity. The average walking speed of the high-intensity group was 3.7 miles per hour, or about 4.3 METs, well below the 6.0-MET definition for high-intensity or vigorous activity. For this group of women, 4.3 METs was high intensity. Many of our clients fall into this overweight, middle-age group, and we have found that as soon as they start to push themselves while walking, they are easily in the moderately vigorous to vigorous level based on perceived exertion and heart rate monitoring.

It's important to help your walking clients understand their effort levels. For many years, health and fitness professionals recommended that people work to get their heart rates into what was known as the target heart rate zone. This zone was calculated using just age or age and resting heart rate. To determine if they were in the target heart rate zone, people had to regularly check their heart rates. It was easy if they had a heart rate monitor, but it was trickier if they had to stop to manually take their pulse.

Over time, research found that using a scale of rate of perceived exertion (RPE) was just as effective and easier to use (table 3.1). The 1 through 10 scale describes effort level by how vigorous a person would describe their physical activity. RPE levels are subjective and different for every individual. Beginners will not have to go as fast to feel that their exertion levels are difficult. As your participants become more fit, they will have to go

TABLE 3.1 **Rates of Perceived Exertion for Walking**

Activity	Rate of perceived exertion (RPE)	Pace	When to suggest it
Inactive	1-2	Barely moving	Not applicable during workout
Easy	3-5	Leisurely stroll	Warm-up or cool-down
Moderate	5-6	Purposeful	Steady-pace walking and recovery intervals
Brisk	6-7	In a bit of a hurry	Steady-pace walking and recovery intervals
Fast	7-8	You're late for an appointment	Longer intervals 60+ sec
Very Fast	8-9	You're trying to catch a bus as it's pulling away	Shorter intervals (e.g., 20-60 sec)
Sprint	10	You're racing for your life	Really short intervals, less than 20 seconds

faster to feel this higher intensity. That's the goal! It shows that the body is becoming better conditioned.

The talk test is another way to teach clients how to self-evaluate for exercise intensity. The talk test simply relates intensity to the ability to talk or even sing. If a person can sing, it's low intensity. At a moderate intensity, conversation is possible but singing is not. When it becomes hard to speak, it's vigorous. Encourage walkers to listen to their bodies and walk at a pace that's appropriate for them for the warm-up, interval drills, recovery phases of interval drills, and the cool-down.

More Ways to Rev Up a Walk

Speed isn't the only way to bump up the intensity of walking. Hills, stairs, and pole walking offer great opportunities to increase the challenge. Adding extra load to the body through added weight is another way to add intensity, although some of these methods can be risky for reasons we will discuss below. You must be sure the benefits outweigh any risks for each client.

Hills

Everyone has experienced the increase in intensity that happens when climbing uphill, whether it's outdoors or on a treadmill. There's no question

Steps to Speed

Here's how to estimate speed based on the number of steps per minute (SPM). These estimates are based on research from University of Massachusetts [18] and Boise State University [20].

100-110 SPM = 2.5 miles per hour = 24 minutes per mile

105-120 SPM = 3.0 miles per hour = 20 minutes per mile

115-130 SPM = 3.5 miles per hour = 17 minutes per mile

125-140 SPM = 4.0 miles per hour = 15 minutes per mile

135-150 SPM = 4.5 miles per hour = 13 minutes per mile

140-155 SPM = 5.0 miles per hour = 12 minutes per mile

that this is a viable way of cranking up the intensity. Depending on the grade of the hill, walking on an incline can elevate calorie burn by about 60 percent without changing speed, according to the *Compendium for Physical Activity*. For every 1 percent increase in grade, calorie burn increases by 12 percent, or about 10 more calories per mile for a 150-pound person. Even if pace slows down on the incline, the cardio workout will be as good as walking briskly on level ground, according to a Colorado State University study [21]. Hilly terrain also provides natural intensity intervals on the uphill and recovery intervals on the downhill. And, hills provide natural strength training. In one study, walking uphill activated three times as many muscle fibers in the glutes compared with walking on level terrain [22]. Since downhills can be tough on the knees and going uphill can encourage poor posture, it's important to teach good hill technique. (See Hill Technique sidebar in chapter 4.)

Stairs

You've probably experienced that huffing and puffing upon reaching the top of a staircase. That's not surprising, considering that stair climbing is twice as taxing as brisk walking on level terrain and 50 percent harder than walking up a steep incline or lifting weights, according to a small Canadian study [23]. And peak exertion was reached much faster when climbing stairs. Stairs can offer a fun and challenging twist to walking workouts. Because they are so strenuous, proceed cautiously, especially with speedy ascents and considering who is in your class. Slow and steady climbs can be just as effective as faster or higher inclines, burning calories two to three times faster than brisk walking on level ground. To build strength, include drills, like taking the steps two at a time. Just make sure that you are teaching good form and remind clients that proper technique is more important than speed on drills like these. To protect the low back from strain, encourage tall posture. For those who already experience low-back issues, keep stair climbing to one at a time. Because going down can be jarring on joints, cue walkers to go slowly, maintain control, and land lightly. A variation to change the plane of motion and work opposing muscles is to have walkers climb the stairs laterally, standing with their feet parallel to the stairs and stepping up. Always remind them to stay to their right as they go up and down the staircase to avoid any collisions.

Nordic Walking

With origins in Finland, Nordic walking utilizes two poles that resemble ski or hiking poles to add an upper-body workout to a walk. Unlike hiking poles that have points to stick into the ground, these poles have rubber tips designed for speed and hand straps that enable more upper-body engagement. On hilly, rocky terrain, hiking poles help with balance and reduce impact during downhill walking, whereas pole walking is usually done on level terrain, and the motion resembles cross-country skiing. The pole is planted behind the body and then used to push off. Studies have shown increases of 20 to 25 percent in cardiovascular load and calorie burn when walking with poles compared to without them. Despite working harder, people using poles tend to report ratings of perceived exertion that are similar to walking without poles. Adding pole walking to your classes can add variety and may be a welcome alternative for walkers who struggle to get faster. But first you'll need training in the technique. The American Nordic Walking Association is a good place to start. Unlike other walking classes, you'll need a plan for the equipment. You can either purchase poles yourself and provide them for classes, or you can require attendees to purchase their own poles. Quality poles cost from $80 to $100 USD.

Considerations for Adding Load

In theory, it makes sense to add weight to walking. The more weight being carried, the harder it will be to walk, resulting in increased intensity and calorie burn. However, in most cases, the risks outweigh the benefits. In fact, we emphatically discourage using dumbbells or ankle weights. Even the benefits of weighted backpacks or vests may not be as great as you think.

Dumbbells

An easy, inexpensive way to add weight is to carry dumbbells while walking. This idea became popular back in the 1980s when foam-covered dumbbells with a strap were created and promoted for walking. Most hand weights designed for walking are one to five pounds—not enough to produce any significant effect. In theory, a person weighing 150 pounds and walking for half an hour at 3.5 miles per hour would burn 153 calories. Carrying five-pound weights (probably more than most people could manage for a half-hour walk), they'd burn an additional 12 calories. That's assuming maintaining pace with the extra weight. The arms act like pendulums, swinging back and forth. The heavier the pendulum, the slower it swings.

Nordic Walking

Case Study

During a career spanning several decades, Barb Gormley, a group fitness leader and personal trainer, has taught almost every fitness class that has made its way into gyms. But one workout has dominated her business for about 15 years now, and that's Nordic walking, sometimes referred to as urban pole walking or urban poling. Barb was coaching a local walking group when Urban Poling sent her a pair of Nordic walking poles to try out and consider for her group. When she used them on her own, she was disappointed because she wasn't getting a better workout than without poles, but that changed when she got coached. A coach from Urban Poling showed her proper technique to engage her abdominal muscles and increase her cardio workout. She not only became a convert to Nordic walking but also a master trainer, certifying coaches in Nordic walking.

Barb offers three levels of pole walking classes each week. A Gentle Beginner class attracts people with limited mobility due to spinal stenosis, recent joint replacements, or cardiac events for example. This 45-minute "stop and start" class encourages taking sitting breaks as needed. The Beginner class is the next step up and may include graduates from the Gentle Beginner class. It lasts for 60 minutes and has fewer breaks. Her All Levels class is a more challenging 60-minute workout for people with a range of fitness abilities. All classes are offered year-round.

Barb has discovered that people stay with the programs for three reasons: They get a good workout, enjoy the social aspect, and get to sightsee while they exercise! To keep classes fresh, she changes the outdoor route and the focus of the workout every class. For example, one workout, she may encourage participants to walk more than 8,500 steps. In another, she may add walking lunges or standing push-ups. A cool-down stretch is always included at the end. Even though all of Gormley's classes are held in one large urban park and one large urban cemetery, she has found that there is much to discover, including a vegetable garden, zoo, ravines, historical spots, and horticultural sights in these spaces that make for interesting destinations and diversions.

For more information, go to www.americannordicwalking.com or www.urbanpoling.com.

When the arms slow down, so do the legs, because the nervous system is wired so that arms and legs are in sync. Even slowing down a little, say to 3.2 miles per hour because of the weights, means the body will burn almost 20 fewer calories than walking normally without weights.

When researchers put this technique for pumping up walking to the test, they found that the only effect of walking while holding a three-pound weight in each hand was an increase in effort. There was no increase in calorie burn compared to when the people walked without weights, even though they were walking at similar paces, according to the study published in the *Journal of Exercise Rehabilitation* [24]. This may seem surprising, but studies of African women who carry much heavier loads on their heads show that alterations in gait minimize the impact on energy expenditure. These women can carry up to 20 percent of their weight (that's 30 pounds for a 150-pound woman) without burning any extra calories than if they were not carrying anything [25].

In addition, swinging extra weight at the end of each arm puts a lot of stress on shoulders, elbows, and wrists and could lead to strained muscles, ligaments, or tendons in these areas. And every pound added increases the impact on joints.

People carrying weights in hopes of getting shapelier arms (or legs by using ankle weights) will get better and faster results by doing strength exercises for those specific areas two or three times a week. Muscles must be challenged to build strength and definition. Think about what people lift and carry during everyday life: bags of groceries; 5- to 10-pound bags of apples, flour, or potatoes while baking or cooking; baskets of clothes and jugs of detergent when doing laundry; suitcases; and children. Swinging a three- to five-pound dumbbell while walking provides no challenge compared to what muscles are used to hauling.

Ankle Weights

We cringe when we hear this suggestion, and we've even seen it made by doctors and researchers. In addition to all the reasons walking with dumbbells is not recommended, walking with ankle weights adds impact to what was once a low-impact, joint-friendly form of exercise—a key driver for many people in choosing walking as their way to work out. And with both dumbbells and ankle weights, loading weight at the end of extremities is completely unnatural. As a result, it can affect biomechanics, leading to problems in other areas of the body, and it will do little if anything to increase strength or improve muscle tone.

Weighted Backpack

There's a movement, including competitive events, around an activity called *rucking*. The name comes from the rucksacks (basically backpacks) that military personnel fill with 100 or more pounds of gear and then carry for training. Since the weight is around the torso instead of at the ends of extremities, there's less risk of injury; however, there's still an increase in impact that could cause problems, especially if the weight is moving around. Some backpacks are specially designed for a snug fit and use flat weights that lay close to the body.

Weighted Vests

Close-fitting vests with pockets for half- or one-pound weights so weight can be easily adjusted are used. This method of weighted walking also has the advantage of placing the extra weight around the torso. Compared to a backpack, the vest better distributes the weight in that area instead of putting it all on the back. Weighted vests have even been used in studies with postmenopausal women and show promise in improving bone density and reducing risk of osteoporosis.

There are a variety of ways to increase walking intensity. However, based on our research and experience, we believe that increasing speed is the most effective. It's been a successful strategy for us in coaching thousands of clients. The next chapter will help you understand how teaching good walking technique sets the foundation for increasing speed while maintaining a low risk for injury.

References

1. Physical Activity Council. 2018. "2018 Participation Report: The Physical Activity Council's Annual Study Tracking Sports, Fitness, and Recreation Participation in the US." www.physicalactivitycouncil.com/pdfs/current.pdf.
2. U.S. Department of Health and Human Services. 2008. "2008 Physical Activity Guidelines for Americans." https://health.gov/paguidelines/pdf/paguide.pdf.
3. U.S. Department of Health and Human Services. 2018. "Physical Activity Guidelines for Americans: 2nd edition." https://health.gov/paguidelines/second-edition/pdf/Physical_Activity_Guidelines_2nd_edition.pdf.
4. Duncan, J.J., Gordon, N.F., and Scott, C.B. 1991. "Women Walking for Health and Fitness. How Much Is Enough?" *Journal of the American Medical Association* 266 (23): 3295-99. www.ncbi.nlm.nih.gov/pubmed/1960829.
5. Manson, J.E., Greenland, P., LaCroix, A.Z., Stefanick, M.L., Mouton, C.P., Oberman, A., Perri, M.G., David S.S., Pettinger, M.B., and Siscovick, D.S. 2002. "Walking Compared With Vigorous Exercise for the Prevention of Cardiovascular Events in Women." *The New England Journal of Medicine* 347: 716-25. www.nejm.org/doi/full/10.1056/NEJMoa021067.
6. Duncan, G.E., Anton, S.D, and Sydeman, S.J. 2005. "Prescribing Exercise at Varied Levels of Intensity and Frequency: A Randomized Trial." *Archives of Internal Medicine* 165 (20): 2362-69. https://jamanetwork.com/journals/jamainternalmedicine/fullarticle/486782.
7. Merlo, C., Sorino, N., Myers, J., Sassone, B., Pasanisi, G., Mandini, S., Guerzoni, F., Napoli, N., Conconi, F., Mazzoni, G., Chiaranda, G., and Grazzi, G. 2018. "Moderate Walking Speed Predicts Hospitalization in Hypertensive Patients With Cardiovascular Disease." *European Journal of Preventive Cardiology* 25 (14): 1558-60. http://journals.sagepub.com/doi/full/10.1177/2047487318767463.
8. Pellikaan, P., Giarmatzis, G., Vander Sloten, J., Verschueren, S., and Jonkers, I. 2018. "Ranking of Osteogenic Potential of Physical Exercises in Postmenopausal Women Based on Femoral Neck Strains." *PLOS One* 13 (4): e0195463. https://journals.plos.org/plosone/article?id=10.1371/journal.pone.0195463.
9. Feskanich, D., Willett, W., and Colditz, G. 2002. "Walking and Leisure-Time Activity and Risk of Hip Fracture in Postmenopausal Women." *Journal of the American Medical Association* 288 (18): 2300-06. https://jamanetwork.com/journals/jama/fullarticle/195504.
10. Young, S.N. 2007. "How to Increase Serotonin in the Human Brain Without Drugs." *Journal of Psychiatry and Neuroscience* 32 (6): 394-99. https://www.ncbi.nlm.nih.gov/pmc/articles/PMC2077351/.

11. Szuhany, K.L., Bugatti, M., and Otto, M.W. 2015. "A Meta-Analytic Review of the Effects of Exercise on Brain-Derived Neurotrophic Factor." *Journal of Psychiatric Research* 60 (1): 56-64. https://www.ncbi.nlm.nih.gov/pmc/articles/PMC4314337/.
12. Brown, J.C., Harhay, M.O., and Harhay, M.N. 2014. "Walking Cadence and Mortality Among Community-Dwelling Older Adults." *Journal of General Internal Medicine* 29 (9): 1263-69. https://link.springer.com/article/10.1007%2Fs11606-014-2926-6.
13. Ainsworth, B.E., Haskell, W.L., Herrmann, S.D., Meckes, N., Bassett, D.R., Tudor-Locke, C., Greer, J.L., Vezina, J., Whitt-Glover, M.C., and Leon, A.S. 2011. "2011 Compendium of Physical Activities: A Second Update of Codes and MET Values." *Medicine & Sciences in Sports & Medicine* 43 (8): 1575-81. www.ncbi.nlm.nih.gov/pubmed/21681120.
14. Greiwe, J.S. and Kohrt, W.M. 2000. "Energy Expenditure During Walking and Jogging." *Journal of Sports Medicine and Physical Fitness* 40 (4): 297-302. www.ncbi.nlm.nih.gov/pubmed/11296999.
15. Schwarz, M., Urhausen, A., Schwarz, L., Meyer, T., and Kindermann, W. 2006. "Cardiocirculatory and Metabolic Responses at Different Walking Intensities." *British Journal of Sports Medicine* 40 (1): 64-7. www.ncbi.nlm.nih.gov/pmc/articles/PMC2491943/?tool=pubmeduy87.
16. Duncan et al. 1991.
17. U.S. Department of Health and Human Services. 2008.
18. Tudor-Locke, T., Agular, E.J., Han, H., Ducharme, S.W., Schuna, J.M., Barreira, T.V., Moore, C.C., Busa, M.A., Lim, J., Sirard, J.R., Chipkin, S.R., Staudenmayer, J. 2019. "Walking Cadence (Steps/Min) and Intensity in 21-40 Year Olds: CADENCE-Adults." *International Journal of Behavioral Nutrition and Physical Activity* 16: 8. https://ijbnpa.biomedcentral.com/track/pdf/10.1186/s12966-019-0769-6.
19. Irving, B.A., Davis, C.K., Brock, D.W., Weltman, J.Y., Swift, D., Barrett, E.J., Gaesser, G.A., and Weltman, A. 2008. "Effect of Exercise Training Intensity on Abdominal Visceral Fat and Body Composition." *Medicine & Science in Sports & Exercise* 40 (11): 1863-72. www.ncbi.nlm.nih.gov/pmc/articles/PMC2730190.
20. Hoeger, W.W.K., Bond, L., Ransdell, L., Shimon, J., and Merugu, S. 2008. "One-Mile Step Count at Walking and Running Speeds." *American College of Sports Medicine's Health and Fitness Journal* 12 (1): 14-19. https://journals.lww.com/acsm-healthfitness/Fulltext/2008/01000/ONE_MILE_STEP_COUNT_AT_WALKING_AND_RUNNING_SPEEDS.7.aspx.
21. Ehlen, K.A., Reiser, R.F., and Browning, R.C. 2011. "Energetics and Biomechanics of Incline Treadmill Walking in Obese Adults." *Medicine & Science in Sports & Exercise* 43 (7): 1251-59. www.ncbi.nlm.nih.gov/pubmed/21200344.
22. Franz, J.R. and Kram, R. 2012. "The Effects of Grade and Speed on Leg Muscle Activations During Walking." *Gait & Posture* 35 (1): 143-47. www.ncbi.nlm.nih.gov/pmc/articles/PMC3262943.
23. Benn, S.J., McCartney, N., and McKelvie, R.S. 1996. "Circulatory Responses to Weight Lifting, Walking, and Stair Climbing in Older Males." *American Journal of the Geriatric Society* 44 (2): 121-25. www.ncbi.nlm.nih.gov/pubmed/8576499.
24. Campana, C.T. and Costa, P.B. 2017. "Effects of Walking With Handheld Weights on Energy Expenditure and Excess Postexercise Oxygen Consumption." *Journal of Exercise Rehabilitation* 13 (6): 641-46. www.ncbi.nlm.nih.gov/pmc/articles/PMC5747198.
25. Maloiy, G.M., Heglund, N.C., Prager, L.M., Cavagna, G.A., and Taylor, C.R. 1986. "Energetic Cost of Carrying Loads: Have African Women Discovered an Economic Way?" *Nature* 319 (6055): 668-69. www.ncbi.nlm.nih.gov/pubmed/3951538.

4

Coach Proper Technique

It's time to transform walking to a workout. Most people have been walking since the time they were about 12 months old. Through those decades of walking, they have developed patterned and recognizable gaits. It is possible to recognize a friend by gait before recognizing the face. Anatomy is partially responsible for this. These patterns are reinforced every time a person walks, creating strong neuropathways from brain to muscle. A message starts in the brain and is sent along a neuropathway to the necessary muscle for activation. This pathway saves the brain energy. It is not necessary to think through every muscle contraction to walk. Any change to walking technique requires patience and repeated reminders to rewrite the neuropathway messaging created over decades of walking.

By way of analogy, let's consider how we brush our teeth every day. Most of us have been brushing our teeth for a long time, and the hand movement pattern is well ingrained in the brain and muscles, just as it is for walking. People typically use the dominant hand to brush teeth. Using the nondominant hand can lead to frustration, and teeth don't feel as clean. We cannot manage the toothbrush with enough dexterity to clean them properly. The great news is that we can change! Over time, we gain skill with our nondominant hand and become as dexterous as with the dominant one. Yeah! Our teeth feel clean again!

Similarly, you can improve walking gait to get an aerobic workout. Making small changes progressively reveals a walking athlete within, and you can help others find their inner athletes.

No matter what the motivating factor responsible for bringing a person to walking class, whether it's a desire to get or stay healthy or lose weight, we should increase cardiorespiratory workouts while minimizing risks for injury. These desires can be met by simply walking as fast as possible without any attention to walking technique, but experience has shown us that the workout will be improved and the risk for injury will be lowered with a walking technique that increases speed and lowers impact.

Good technique makes walking an accessible and sustainable workout with greater benefits and fewer injuries than would be achieved by simply picking up the pace from a strolling gait.

Using our knowledge of the muscles required to power the walking gait, let's take a fresh look at how to coach people so they recruit those muscles.

Sound Steps

Case Study

It's a natural fit for parks and recreation departments to offer walking programs like Seattle's Sound Steps, a free, volunteer-supported walking and hiking program designed to increase physical activity and social connections. Organized under the auspices of the city's Lifelong Recreation program and targeted at the population older than 50, the program offers weekly walks of varying degrees of difficulty throughout the city in neighborhoods, parks, and even the zoo. Most of the weekly walks are free. Monthly hikes, for various levels, are offered for a fee that includes transportation to the trailheads. For beginners, those with mobility issues, or those needing assistive devices, there are walks at a local mall. There are also options for walking laps indoors to music. There's something for everyone, with walks as short as a half mile or as long as five or six miles. There is also fun to be had at seasonal events, such as a holiday lights walk that includes a potluck dinner.

Those looking for a challenge can join the annual spring training program. Building fitness through increasingly long walks, participants train for the culminating event choosing either a 5K or half marathon distance. They receive a training schedule with suggestions for three weekly walks on their own, as well as a supported group walk on Saturdays.

Success of the program depends on volunteer leaders and spreading the word. Leaders are typically age-peers from the community. Undergraduate students studying public health promotion provide support in a unique intergenerational relationship. Both students and older adults report enjoying the opportunity to share experiences and develop relationships with a demographic with whom they do not regularly interact. Looking toward the future, program coordinator Tamara Keefe says the goals are to build attendance at currently scheduled walk locations and meet the needs of underserved populations by supporting program growth in areas of the city not currently represented.

For more information, go to www.seattle.gov/parks/find/sound-steps-(50).

This technique will focus on four progressions to improve posture, stride length, muscle recruitment, foot placement, and more. Yes, it's time to rethink walking.

The progressions are designed as a step-wise process to help clients feel successful immediately. Begin with simple gait refinement, moving to greater and more complex muscle recruitment as well as improvement in body awareness. From the first progression, walkers will improve speed. Subsequent progressions will introduce new techniques and refine them further to lead to greater speed and a more vigorous workout while minimizing injury risks. When introducing these progressions, always respect your clients' abilities to work within the constraints of their anatomy.

Progression 1: Eyes Up, Elbows Bent

The first progression focuses on the position and movement of the upper body. While it specifically addresses the head and arms, good upper-body posture is an important topic to teach to all walkers. If you stop and observe people as they walk, you'll see a variety of postures, such as bending at the waist or sinking into the pelvis, all of which inhibit a powerful walking stride. Progression 1 (figure 4.1) addresses postural challenges to fast walking, a good workout, and our intention to lower risk for injury.

Eyes Up

Look to the horizon so the chin is parallel to the ground. Encourage clients to look to where they are going. The anatomical effect is to immediately stack the ears over shoulders and the center of gravity. This small, yet powerful, change to spine alignment creates excellent posture. A strong walk begins with good posture. When walkers stand tall, they open their chests, making it easier to breathe. They lift out of the pelvis, allowing their legs to swing more freely.

As simple as this revision is, some people need constant reminders to lift the head and look ahead. This is not surprising since so many daily activities encourage a hunched, shoulders-rounded posture—sitting at a computer, driving in a car, texting on a phone, even cooking or reading a book. It is a challenge to change years of neurological and muscle memory. Moreover, some walkers are fearful of tripping and falling. They do not trust that their peripheral vision is sufficient to see obstacles that might make them stumble.

For clients who are too fearful to look at the horizon or are walking in areas with a lot of obstacles, encourage them to instead look 10 to 20 feet in front of them. This will bring their heads up and allow them to spot hazards in time to react. One client, along with her family, was brought to tears when she discovered this technique.

When Marion came to a class with her daughters, she was a spunky 74-year-old who'd been walking regularly for 12 years despite having Parkinson's disease. During the single-session class, everyone did a timed lap at the beginning and end so they could see how they improved after adding technique to their walking. We had never had a client who was slower on their final lap until Marion. But as she approached the group at the finish line, she cheered with a smile, "I did better!" and began crying tears of joy. She explained that for the first time in three years, she was able to walk and look at the trees. As the disease had progressed, she had started to look down at her feet because she was fearful of falling. But at the suggestion of looking just 10 to 20 feet in front of her, Marion felt confident enough to lift her head up, and now she enjoys walking even more as she takes in the scenery.

The posture improvement alone is a great take-home benefit for your clients. Many people look and feel better when they stand tall. And it often

Walk Fast to Live Longer

The faster people walk as they age, the longer they may live. People over age 65 who naturally walk at 2.2 miles per hour or faster tend to live longer than expected based on their age and gender, according to research [2]. Those walking 1.3 miles per hour or slower were at greater risk for an early death.

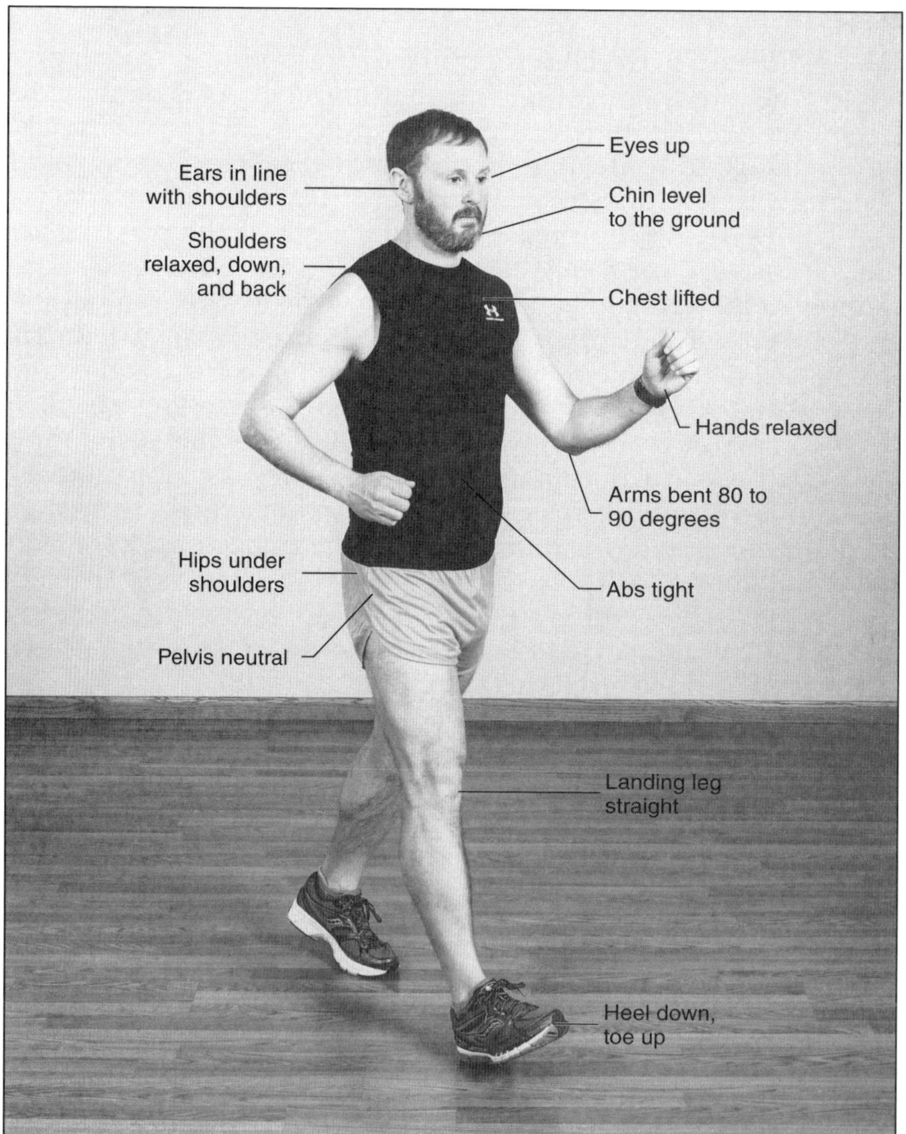

FIGURE 4.1 Keep these pointers in mind as you coach good walking posture.

shows. Clients have said that friends or coworkers have commented that they look like they've lost weight even when they haven't. Good posture also allows for more effective recruitment of the muscles in the posterior chain, which we will talk about in a later progression.

To help develop good posture, instruct your clients to imagine a string attached to the top of their heads that is lifting or stretching them while their feet remain on the ground. You can illustrate the effect this has by having them place their thumbs on their lowest rib and their index fingers on the top of their pelvic bone as they stand normally (figure 4.2). Then tell them to feel the string lifting and stretching them. As they do this, have them pay attention to how the space between their rib cage and pelvis elongates. These are simple strategies that you can encourage your clients to practice outside of class, anytime they are walking.

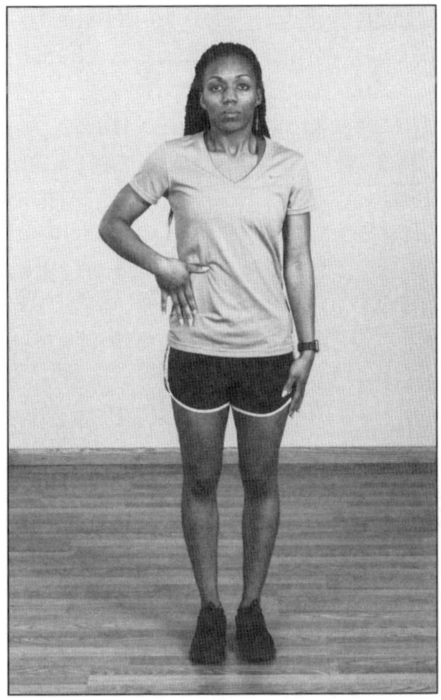

FIGURE 4.2 Place the thumb on the lowest rib and the index finger on the top of the pelvic bone. When standing up tall, the space will expand compared to when posture is slouchy.

To teach good posture in class, find a wall that is taller than your tallest class participant. Have everyone remove water belts or packs. Get them to stand with their backs to the wall: heels, glutes, shoulder blades, and backs of their heads against the wall. This aligns the ears, shoulders, and hips in excellent posture. Have them stand there to appreciate the work that goes into keeping a tall posture (which means those muscles need strengthening)! Encourage them by saying it is easier to maintain this alignment while moving.

Elbows Bent

The second part of progression 1, with its focus on upper-body position and movement, encourages walkers to bend their arms at the elbow the way they would if they were running. Humans do this instinctively when they run because the brain understands the physics of the situation: The arm is a lever, and a shorter lever is easier to move more quickly than a longer lever. Visualize this by imagining a metronome. To increase its cadence, you move the weight closer to the fixed end (fulcrum) around which the lever pivots. To slow it down, you move the weight farther from the pivot point. When breaking into a run, most people bend their arms so that the weight of the arm is closer to the fulcrum, which in the human body is the shoulder, making it easier to go faster.

Oddly, human intuition to bend the elbow and shorten the arm length doesn't kick in when most people try to walk more quickly. More often, they will break into a run rather than bend their arms and stick with the walking gait. For those who want to keep walking but increase speed, bending the arms is essential. As the arm lever shortens, it takes less effort to swing the arms, and they swing faster. Because the brain always keeps the swinging of the arms and legs synchronized, increasing the cadence (speed) of the arms results in increased leg cadence. The faster the arms swing, the faster the legs will go.

Here are the key instructions to ensure a proper arm swing.

Bend the Elbows 80 to 90 Degrees

Encourage walkers to position their arms the way they would when running. They should maintain this bent position throughout the entire range of motion (figure 4.3). A helpful cue is to imagine the bent arm in a cast so it cannot be straightened, and the swinging motion should come from the shoulders only. As you observe your clients, keep an eye out for elbow extension as their arms swing backward. We call this common mistake "drumstick arms" because it's like striking a drum each time the arm is lowered. Help your clients recognize this problem by having them drape a strap around their necks and hold an end in each hand. If they keep their elbows bent, they won't notice the strap on their neck. However, if they extend their arms on the backswing, the strap will slide back and forth across the backs of their necks.

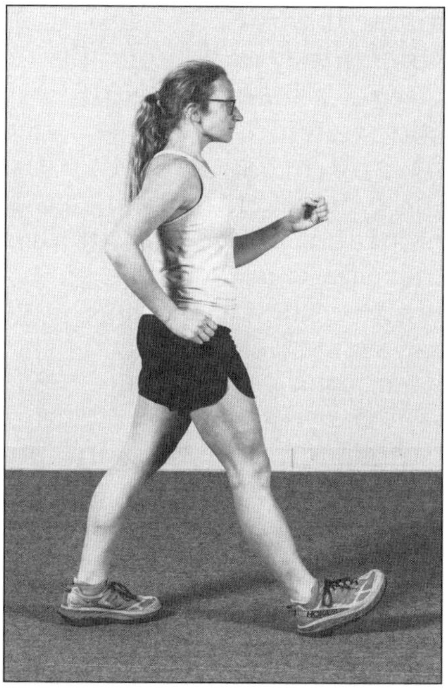

FIGURE 4.3 Bend arms 80 to 90 degrees.

Swing Forward and Back

Walking is a sagittal plane motion (forward and back), so the arms should follow, with the hands making an arc from chest height to hip. If the head is lifted and the eyes are focused forward as the bent arm swings, the hand moving forward should just come into the lower peripheral vision. For an anatomical marker, instruct walkers to swing the arm no higher than chest height (figure 4.4). Imagine a shelf extending out from the chest and keep hands from hitting it. Another image that may help control an overly aggressive arm swing is to picture a headlight on each hand that must keep shining ahead to light the way. If they swing too high, it will shine up to the sky. If they drop their wrists or extend their elbows on the backswing, the light will be directed down toward the ground or behind them. These are important cues because a common tendency is to exaggerate the forward swing. Pumping the hand too far forward can result in the legs following with a long stride in front of the body, which is not an ideal way to improve speed, as you'll learn in progression 2. Also, if the hands are sent upward, energy is being misdirected up rather than forward.

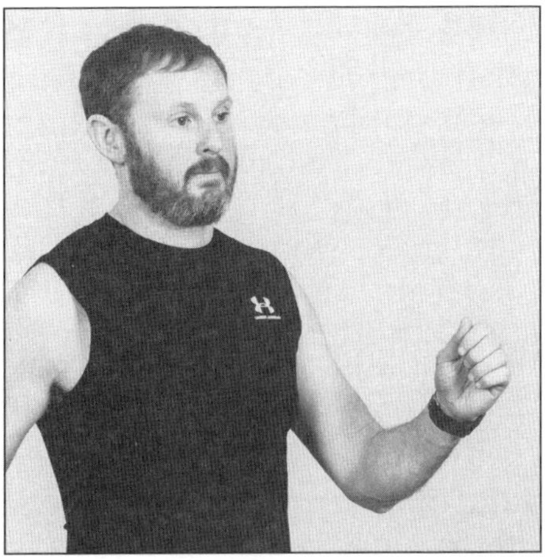

FIGURE 4.4 Swing arm forward to about chest height but no higher.

On the flip side, many walkers downplay the backswing, barely getting their elbows behind their bodies. When a person is properly swinging the arms for maximum power, the hand should graze the hip bone (figure 4.5).

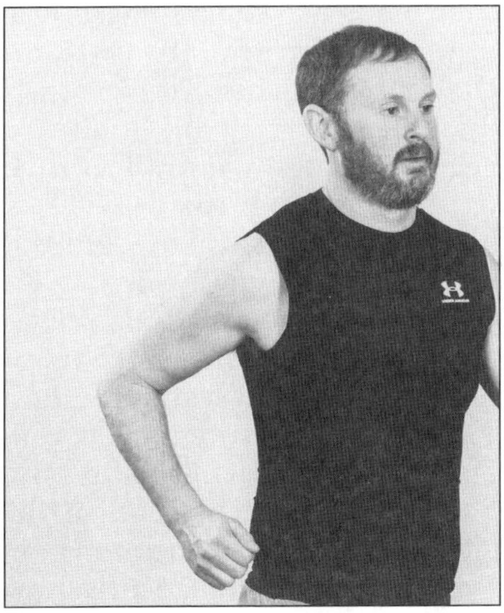

FIGURE 4.5 Swing arm back until the hand is by the hip.

Streamline Movements

Because the shoulder is a multiaxial ball-and-socket joint, arm movement in the sagittal plane includes some rotation. The more aerodynamic a walker's movements, the faster they will go with less effort. The slight rotation that occurs with walking is visible as the arms cross in front of the body. As a coach, be on the lookout for excessive rotation through the torso and discourage clients from allowing their hands to cross the body's midline.

Other common mistakes that compete with the forward motion of walking are allowing the elbows to swing out to the sides like chicken wings or swinging the arms side to side in front of the body. Remind your clients to keep their elbows in and to swing forward and back, not side to side.

Keep Hands Active but Relaxed

Most people will find a naturally comfortable position for fingers and hands, usually either cupped (figure 4.6) or extended like a handshake (figure 4.7). In either position, the hand should be aligned with the wrist, no flexion. Clenched fists are a common mistake. This isometric contraction in the hand and forearm wastes valuable energy and may contribute to tension all the way up the arm and into the neck and upper back. To encourage clients to relax their hands while maintaining a cupped position, have them open their hands so their fingertips are touching their thumbs instead of their palms. Then, tell them to imagine that they are holding an egg, and if they apply too much pressure, it will break.

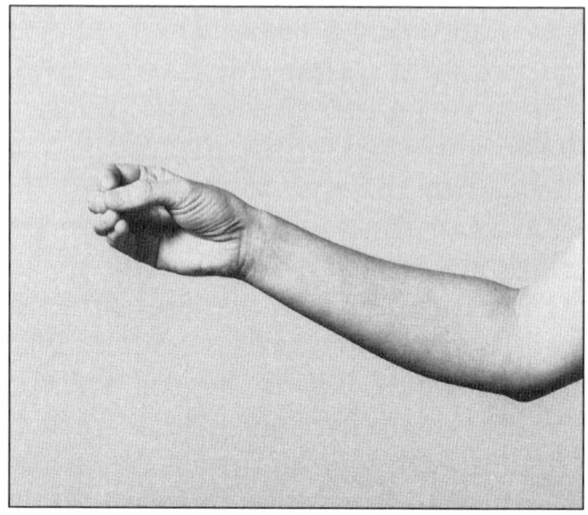

FIGURE 4.6 If hands are clenched, encourage a cupped hand with the fingertips touching the thumb instead of the palm.

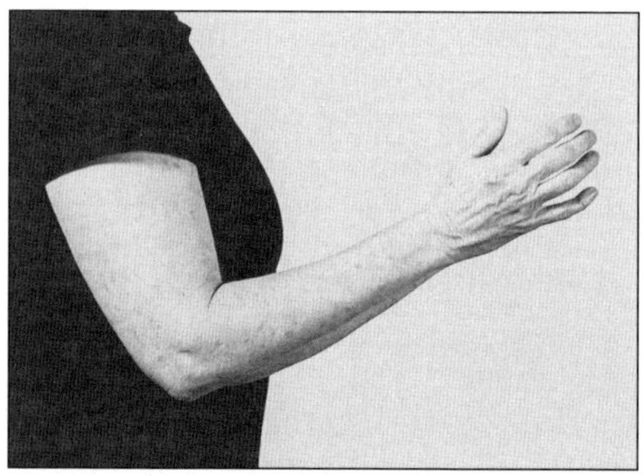

FIGURE 4.7 If hands are limply flexed at the wrist, encourage a handshake position instead.

Other walkers might hold their hands limp from the wrist. This flexion at the wrist usually is accompanied by arms that are not working to the fullest potential. If you see this "limp wrist" in walkers, encourage them to align their hands with their wrists as if they are going to shake someone's hand. Get them to visualize the power that is in the arms. Harnessing arm power will be addressed more completely in progression 3, so it may be best to simply suggest the handshake position to see if that improves the hand position. If it does not, cues associated with progression 3 may result in a change in this hand position.

As walkers add a bent-arm swing to their technique, remind them to keep their shoulders down, back, and relaxed. A common mistake is to pull them up toward their ears as they focus on trying to make all the adjustments. You may also notice this shrugging posture on cold or windy days. Offer friendly cues as needed.

Progression 2: Short, Quick Steps

Our second progression addresses the position and movement of the lower body.

If you had to guess which one of us—Michele at 5'8" or Lee at 5'6"—is speedier, you'd probably pick Michele. Most people think taller people with longer legs can walk faster (Michele hears this all the time), which is reasonable. But the truth is, the shorter person can be faster than the taller one, and this isn't an anomaly. The gold medalist in the women's 20K (12.4 miles) racewalk at the 2016 Olympics stands at only 5'3" tall and averaged a seven-minute-per-mile pace while walking, beating out many taller competitors.

The key to moving faster isn't bigger steps; it's a quicker step cadence. Progression 2 focuses on getting the feet and legs to move more quickly while minimizing impact.

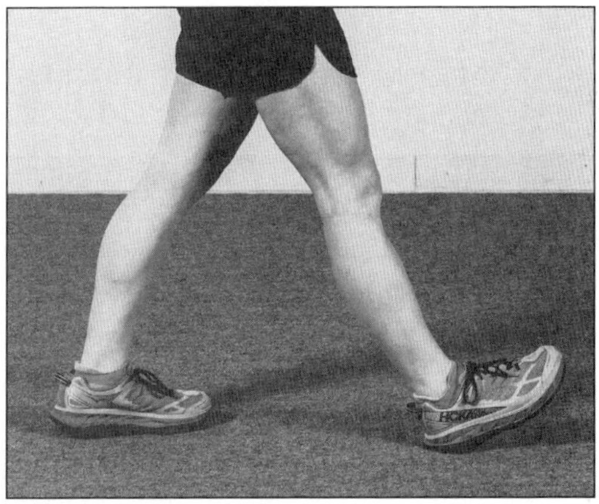

FIGURE 4.8 With the leg farther out in front of the body, it is more work to support and move the COM over the front leg.

Take Short Steps

The significant change in this progression is a shortening of the stride in front of the body. This is done by placing the heel of the landing foot just in front of the body, ahead of the COM. This position minimizes the effort required to push the weight of the body over the front foot. The farther out in front of the body the foot is placed, the more effort it takes to bring the opposite foot forward. Walking has been described as a series of forward falls [3]. But when the leg is extended far out in front of the body (figure 4.8) it acts like a brake, decreasing speed and creating a bouncy, choppy stride that increases impact to the joints in the lower body, especially the knee. When the foot instead lands closer to the body (figure 4.9), there is less impact, and it is easier to roll body mass over the front foot and swing the back foot forward to catch the body as it falls forward onto the next step.

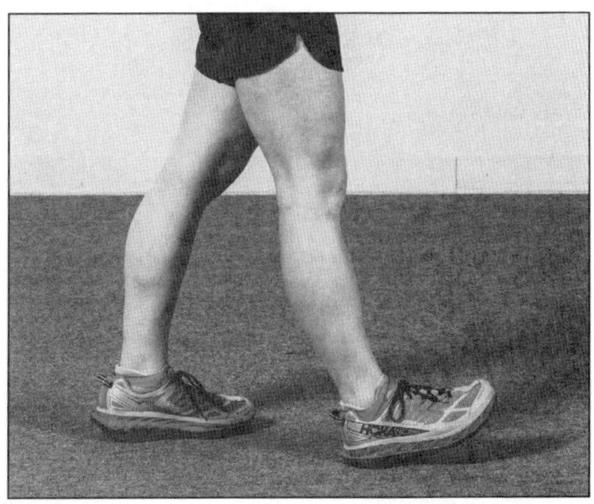

FIGURE 4.9 When the foot lands closer to the body, the COM is more supported, and it takes less effort to move it over the front leg.

This small change to foot placement is remarkably challenging for many people. They are accustomed to what an aerobic walk feels like, and it usually involves a longer stride. Encourage patience with the shorter stride, even though many describe it as feeling like baby steps.

Here are three ways to help your walkers see how short their forward steps should be:

Option 1

- Have walkers press their heels, glutes, shoulder blades, and backs of heads against a wall (remove any waist packs or water bottle holders).
- Identify this as the walking posture (it is easier to maintain while moving).
- Maintaining the line of the body from ankle to crown of the head, let the body fall forward away from the wall.
- As soon as both heels peel off from the ground, step one foot forward to stop the fall. *Note:* The goal is not to wait as long as possible to break the fall. Lift and place the front landing foot as soon as both heels start to peel off the ground.
- The place where the foot lands shows an ideal stride length.

Option 2

- Stand on a level surface, feet together, and hold on to a wall, tree, railing, or back of a bench with one hand for balance.
- Raise one knee up to hip height, the foot of that leg dangling below.
- Lower the heel of that dangling foot straight down to the ground, not back to the starting position.
- This is about the size of the step forward, about three to five inches, that should be taken.

Option 3

- Start by taking big steps and feel the bouncing in the body.
- Then take itty-bitty steps, like kids do at the pool when they are running and the lifeguard yells at them to walk.
- Then go back to the long, bouncy strides.
- Feel the difference?
- Now, shorten the stride until the bouncing is eliminated and stick with that.

If you notice any of your walkers bouncing while they walk, the stride has lengthened to the more familiar higher-impact gait, and they have probably slowed down. Remind them to shorten steps in front of the body. You'll give this cue frequently when leading walking groups.

Land on the Heel

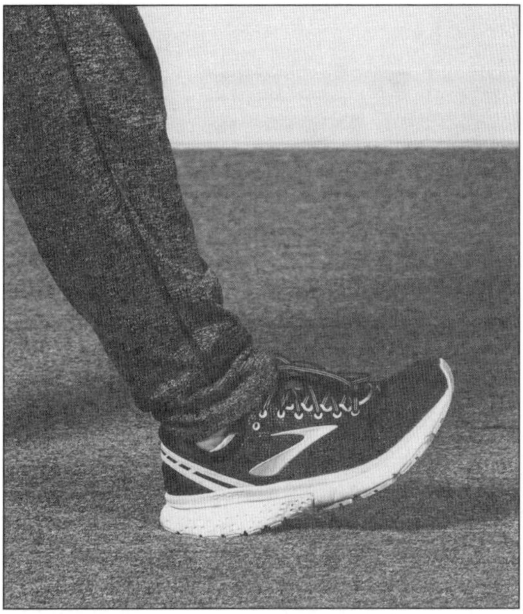

FIGURE 4.10 As the front leg steps forward, land on the heel, pulling the toes up toward the shin.

A key feature of the walking gait is landing with the toes of the front foot up and the heel down (figure 4.10). While directing walkers' focus to heel placement, it's helpful to encourage awareness to range of motion around the ankle. Good range of motion at the ankle as the front heel strikes results in good positioning of the entire leg. The knee of that landing leg is in extension so that the leg looks straight to the observer. If the foot lands flat or on the forefoot, the knee is in flexion and the walk turns into a shuffle or possibly a jog. Heel-down and toe-up foot placement facilitates a smooth heel-to-toe roll that maximizes the range of motion at the ankle. For people with knee injuries or weakness, an emphasis on knee extension builds strength in the quadriceps muscles, helping to stabilize the joint and protect it from injury. Also, a straight-leg landing lowers the risk for knee injury because the braking load of landing is distributed throughout the entire leg rather than in the knee ligaments, as happens when a bent knee takes more impact while running or jogging.

A side effect of increasing step cadence is that walkers often feel shin fatigue, which they will describe as shin pain, even shin splints. It is uncommon for walkers to get shin splints, but the shin fatigue they experience from increasing the cadence can be debilitating and extremely uncomfortable. Encourage them by telling them that this muscular fatigue pain typically decreases over time as they become stronger and familiar with the new technique. See Ease Shin Pain section later in this chapter for ways to help your clients.

Progression 3: Think Back to Move Forward

The third progression emphasizes recruitment of the muscles in the posterior chain of both the upper and lower body. Bringing awareness to the power of the large muscles in the posterior chain is like adding a jet-pack on the back to push the body forward. It radically energizes any walk.

Typically, the muscles in the back of the body are much larger than opposing anterior muscles. Yet most people focus on using the muscles

Ease Shin Pain

Coaching Tip

The most common complaint walkers have when they try to go faster is that their shins burn or hurt. This usually happens because the small muscles in the front of the shins—including the tibialis anterior—are working harder than usual to keep the toes up as the heel lands with every step. Feeling this burn in the shins probably means they are doing something right. As long as the pain subsides upon slowing down, it's usually due to muscle fatigue. (If pain doesn't go away when they slow down or stop walking, they should check with their doctor.) The good news is that the pain will decrease as shins get stronger. In the meantime, here are some strategies to ease the ache.

- **Go in reverse.** If you are walking in a safe area, turn around and take a few backward steps. Walking backward can be a quick way to relieve shin pain. When it subsides, face forward and gradually build back up to the fast pace.
- **Slow down and stretch.** If slowing the pace doesn't alleviate the pain enough, encourage them to stop and do some simple stretches. Lift one foot off the ground at a time and rotate the foot clockwise and counterclockwise. Then, point and flex the foot. Repeat several times until you're ready to start walking again.
- **Increase ankle range of motion.** Tight shin and calf muscles can contribute to problems. For greater ankle flexibility, make sure that these areas are stretched after every walk. (See chapter 6, Shin Area.)
- **Strengthen.** The muscles alongside the shins will get stronger as your walkers do more fast walking, but they can help that process along by adding some shin-strengthening exercises (chapter 7) to their routine.
- **Squeeze the butt as the heel touches the ground.** This progression 3 technique activates the glutes and shortens the stride so that shin muscles don't have to work so hard. This will require concentration on the glutes to do this, which may help distract from the discomfort in the shins.

in the front of the body—punching forward with their arms and reaching out with the front leg—likely because our eyes can see our anterior muscles, see what these muscles are doing, and see where we are going. Our brain makes decisions and sends messages based on that information from our eyes. It is natural to focus on sending the arms and legs forward. By focusing on forward movement of the upper and lower body, the brain sends action messages to smaller anterior muscles. Walkers are going to be limited by the power of smaller muscles to propel them forward, which ultimately limits the workout that can be achieved. Let's get your clients to use their brains to send messages to the larger muscles in the back of the body. These larger muscles function automatically during the walking gait but by visualizing them and actively sending messages to them to work harder, the walking workout is ramped up.

As one arm swings forward, the other arm moves back. As one leg swings forward when walking, the other one pulls back. Instead of directing attention to the forward movement and hence contraction of anterior muscle groups, think about the larger muscles of the posterior chain to drive the motion of the arm swinging back and the opposite leg pulling back. As walkers focus on a powerful backward drive with one arm, the "equal and opposite" reaction is for the other arm to swing forward. In this way, the powerful backswing results in a quick forward movement. This works in the same way for the legs. As one leg is powerfully pulled back, the "equal and opposite" reaction of the other leg is to swing forward quickly.

Drive Elbows Back Instead of Punching Forward

Because our eyes watch our arms move forward, it is tempting to punch them forward when trying to create a more powerful stride. When hitting a punching bag in front of the body, the anterior muscles of the upper body (especially the pectoralis and deltoids) are recruited. These are smaller muscles than the opposing muscles in the back. Walkers can get much more power from the arms by visualizing "elbowing" back. This changes recruitment from anterior muscles to posterior muscles, including the rhomboids and latissimus dorsi. Encourage walkers to visualize pulling the elbow back rather than punching the hand forward. Then let the arm swing forward in a relaxed manner, without forcing or powering it forward.

To teach powerful arm movement, have walkers stand in place and swing their bent arms as they would while walking. Explain that the goal of this exercise is to understand the power of the mind! They will maintain this "arm walk" while changing how their brain visualizes the movement. First, imagine a punching bag directly in front of the body. The brain tells the hand to punch the bag while simultaneously making a mental note of the power behind that punch. Then, with arms still moving, imagine someone is standing a little too close for comfort behind you. The brain tells the elbow to hit back toward that person, making a mental note of the power behind that movement. Most people will feel significantly more powerful in forcefully directing the elbow back rather than punching the hand forward.

Activate the Glutes

Increase power in the lower body by being mindful of the role the glute muscles play in bringing the landing leg back and behind. Just as it is common to power the arms forward to get faster, it is typical for walkers to throw their legs forward to get a longer stride and more speed. Unfortunately, it is easier to get walkers to embrace the pull-back with their arms than it is to get them to recruit the glute muscles. Many people cannot consciously activate their glute muscles, and it is extremely difficult to practice alternating glute contraction at the outset of learning this new walking technique because it happens so quickly. It has been our practice as coaches to ask walkers to do the easier thing, which is to squeeze both glutes at the same time while walking. This effectively powers the leg moving back and gently slows the forward swing of the opposite leg. The contracted glute of the forward-moving leg shortens the forward swing and stride, which is part of our emphasis described earlier in the second progression. As walkers become adept at this, you can introduce drills that encourage deliberate alternating recruitment of these muscles (see One-Leg Propulsion drill in chapter 5). Constantly squeezing the glute muscles can be tiring and counterproductive over time, but at the outset, it helps give walkers the sense of using the largest and most powerful muscles in the legs to power their walk.

Here are two ideas for teaching the gluteal contraction of the walking gait.

1. Standing with the feet under the hips, have walkers place the right foot forward in the heel strike position. Tell them to place their right hand on the right gluteus maximus and pull the leg back, keeping it straight. Encourage them to locate the squeezing contraction of the glute muscle as the leg is pulled back, noting that the instruction given was to "pull the leg back" not "squeeze the glute." The brain understands that to move the leg behind the body, the glute muscle must contract. We can use our brains to more consciously activate these glute muscles during the walk.
2. Standing with the feet under the hips, place the right hand on the right glute and the left hand on the left glute. Ask participants to squeeze the right glute only. Then, squeeze the left glute only. Contract both at the same time. For most people, squeezing both will be easiest. Alternating the glute squeeze is tricky for the brain as a conscious process. We encourage people who are new to this altered walking style to walk squeezing both glutes. This promotes power in the leg moving backward and shortens the stride of the leg moving forward (acting as an assist to the cues we have already given about shortening the stride leg out in front of the body).

Progression 4: Hip Rotation

The fourth progression refines the walking gait to enhance speed and lower injury risk further. As walkers can incorporate the posterior muscle recruitment described in progression three, they get faster to where we have found they describe their gait beginning to feel "robotic" or "peg-legged." While they have discovered the power in their body to propel themselves forward, the resulting speed increase makes them feel like it would be easier and more efficient to run instead of continuing to walk. This is a sweet spot, where calorie burn is high. But it can be problematic if the joints experience an awkwardness that leads to discomfort and possibly injury.

The solution is to introduce your walkers to hip rotation—a movement that makes the gait similar to racewalking. While it may look like the side-to-side hip shaking seen on the dance floor, it is actually a forward and back motion in the sagittal plane. Hip rotation pulls the pelvis back to assist the extension that is happening at the hip as the leg moves back behind. And then as the leg swings forward, the hip follows. One of the images that can help walkers to understand and feel what is happening is to think of their legs extending all the way up to the rib cage. Muscles such as the psoas major are used for walking and attach the legs to the spine, crossing the hip joint. So, as each leg goes forward and then back, the corresponding hip follows.

Hip rotation also engages the oblique abdominal muscles. Just as it was difficult to consciously alternate contraction of the glute muscles, actively engaging the oblique abdominal muscles on alternating sides to bring the pelvis and hip back and forth is tricky. The easiest way to coach this change in walk movement is to have walkers imagine they are walking a narrow plank (about 1.5 times the width of their foot). Bring the heel of the front landing foot to that plank. This automatically forces the abdominals to engage even more strongly than when the foot lands directly under the hip, facilitating the hip rotation we are seeking. You can demonstrate the change by having your clients watch you from behind as you walk normally and then bring your feet closer as if you are walking on a plank. If they have trouble seeing the difference, tie a shirt around your waist to show the swinging more easily. Remind walkers to keep their front legs straight but not locked from the time their heels touch the ground until their feet are underneath them. This leg position also assists in bringing the hip back and protects against injury (see tips later in this chapter).

The positive effect of bringing hip rotation into the walking technique is to engage the oblique abdominals of the core. Many people suffer from low-back injury and pain. Improving core strength is a known antidote. Also, using more core strength through hip rotation will lower the impact felt by the heels, knees, and hips. Without any hip rotation, people trying to get faster simply by speeding up the gait will eventually come to a point where the heel strike happens quickly and with great impact. Transferring the work load to the abdominal muscles in moving the pelvis lowers this impact.

Another great benefit is that the stride becomes lengthened *behind* the body and its center of gravity, moving the toe push-off to a position where it offers greater mechanical advantage. Imagine walking up to a swinging door that is fixed on one side only with hinges. It is common to open that door by pushing as far away from the hinged connection as possible because that is where the least force is required. In other words, pushing opposite the hinges makes the door easier to swing open. Now, imagine the center of gravity of the body like that hinged attachment point of the door, then a toe push-off happening farther away from that point will have greater impact on pushing the body forward, just as pushing the door farther from the hinged side has greater impact on opening the door.

Here are four tips for teaching hip rotation.

1. Because hip rotation happens automatically when the feet land on an imaginary narrow plank, demonstrate to the class. Have them gather behind you as you walk using all the techniques from progressions 1 through 3, with your feet landing on the ground under your hips. After a few moments, change the landing of your feet, positioning them to land on that narrow plank. Do this twice: The first time have them notice your foot placement, and the second time have them notice the resulting change to hip movement. Ask everyone to practice this method, hands on either side of the waist, to feel the resulting abdominal engagement.
2. Stand with the feet close together and place a hand on each hip. Keeping feet and upper torso stationary, pull the right hip back, allowing the left hip to go forward. The right leg will straighten and pull back while the left one will bend forward. Just make sure the hips, not the legs, are driving the action. Most hips will only move an inch or so back and forth.
3. While walking, allow the feet to cross the midline of the body (like a runway model). Place hands between the bottom of the rib cage and the top of the hip bones to feel how the abs are working and the hips are rotating. Then walk normally to compare: transition to a normal walk where the feet aren't crossing the midline but hip movement is maintained. This is a good exercise to practice during your warm-up and cool-down.
4. Remind walkers to gradually introduce hip rotation to their walking technique and to shorten their stride as they do to reduce their risk of injury. As the hip pulls back, it brings the top of the tensor fasciae latae, a muscle that runs down the outside of the thigh, with it. Because the tensor fasciae latae attaches just below the knee, overuse or an exaggerated stride could result in pulling the knee out of alignment.

This progressive approach to walking technique has helped thousands of walkers improve workouts by increasing speed, minimizing risk for injury, and offering them a sense of accomplishment. Walk the walk! By simply implementing the first progression, you and your clients will pick up the pace and get the heart pumping to increase the intensity of a walk. Cardiorespiratory challenge increases as the second, third, and fourth progressions are introduced wherever and whenever possible. Some people will be able to incorporate all progressions almost immediately.

To most effectively coach your walkers, know your audience. Sometimes it is good to teach all progressions in one or two classes; other times, it

Hill Technique

All four progressions come into play with varying emphasis depending on whether you are walking uphill or downhill. Both inclines and declines require an exaggeration of the short stride, making it even shorter than on flat ground.

When heading up a hill, the body automatically leans into the hill, and too often people bend at the waist to manage the lean. Minimize that lean by looking up the hill, lifting the ribcage, and practicing shorter steps. These shorter steps allow the heel to land instead of the sole or ball of the foot. The landing leg should be straight as described in progression 2, but this is not always possible, depending on the grade of the hill. If the hill gets very steep, a slight bend in the knee is acceptable but continue pulling the toes up to land on the heels. A flat foot landing will act as a brake at each step.

Heading downhill, keep the legs as straight as possible, with foot placement on the narrow plank that was taught in the fourth progression. Maintain a straight leg until the foot passes underneath and behind the hip. This requires considerable mobility through the hips and waist and results in hip rotation. Teaching downhill technique is a great opportunity to help walkers access hip rotation, keeping in mind that people may not have the mobility and flexibility in their hips to accomplish it right away, so landing with a slight bend in the knee is an acceptable alternative. Because it is difficult to get an aerobic workout walking downhill and because there is considerable opportunity to get injured (just as with running), encourage a slow pace that allows a focus on form, especially the techniques of the fourth progression. A bobbing head is a good indicator that more technique cues should be given when practicing uphill and downhill walking.

is helpful to teach one progression a week. It is always good to return to the progressions on a regular basis during walking workout classes. Spend one class where, during all speed intervals, people will focus on pulling the arms back. In another class, focus on pulling the toes of the landing leg up.

Know that everyone will experience greatest success when they can remain relaxed, finding ease in the changes they make to their walking gait. Remind them to focus on one small change at a time, trusting that eventually it will all come together.

Good walking technique often results in faster walking without much effort, and it is the starting place for injury-free power walking. The next step is to ask them to go fast intentionally during drills. Our next chapter is filled with ideas for creating effective walking workouts based on sound physiological principles and the latest research on interval training.

What About the Toe Push-Off?

Coaching Tip

If you've done any previous reading about walking technique, you may be wondering why none of the four progressions address the toe push-off. It is an important component of the walking gait—land on the heel, roll through the foot, and push off with the toes. In addition, activating a strong toe push-off can increase speed, and this action is a key component of racewalking. But our typical clients are not typical racewalkers.

When Lee started coaching, she instructed the toe push-off, but the more people she coached, the more she realized that they were underutilizing larger muscles that could also impact speed. In addition, the most common complaints she heard from clients were about foot issues, such as bunions, Morton's neuromas, and flat feet. During the push-off, there is increased pressure on the metatarsal arch. Lee started to worry that as people focused more on the toe push-off, it may result in too much pressure on the vulnerable, small muscles, tendons, and ligaments in the metatarsal arch, especially for those carrying extra weight. Instead, Lee has coached walkers to reach speeds of up to six miles per hour by recruiting larger muscles in the body, which is the focus of the four progressions, without emphasizing the toe push-off. Although we're not aware of any research to support Lee's experience, it made sense to stick with that coaching hierarchy based on her success.

But that doesn't mean that you should ignore the toe push-off. Lee has used it with clients who have worked through all four progressions successfully and are looking for the next tweak to their form that will improve performance. Michele also uses it when she feels that clients need variety, and she's found it helpful when trying to get clients to lengthen stride length behind them.

To teach a proper push-off, start by helping clients understand exactly when the push-off is happening. The heel strikes the ground, and then the foot rolls through to the toe push-off. As they roll forward and come up onto the toes of what is now the back foot, the upper body is passing over the top of the front foot as it moves behind. Walking up a hill is a good opportunity to feel this action. The key to getting maximum acceleration from the push-off is to wait until the toes are well behind the body. Mark Fenton, former coach of the US racewalking team and researcher at the Olympic Training Center's Sports Science Laboratory in Colorado Springs, Colorado, offers this tip: Think about keeping the toes on the ground as long as possible as the heel lifts, so someone walking behind you can see as much of the sole of the shoe as possible. This will extend the stride length more behind the body than in front. If the back foot is too close under the pelvis, the toe push-off will propel the body up instead of forward.

Another way to achieve a longer stride length behind the body and to delay the toe push-off as long as possible is to maintain a straight leg for as long as possible. If calf muscles are tight, the heel will peel off the ground prematurely. Stretching these muscles will allow the heel to stay in contact with the ground longer and increase the stride length behind the body.

PART III

WALKING WORKOUTS

5

Design Effective Workouts

Look at the list of programs and services for any gym, community center, or worksite fitness facility, and you're likely to see a dizzying array of group exercise classes, from basic cardio dance, Spinning, and kickboxing to creative combinations like Pilates and boxing, treadmill running and strength training, and cardio and drumming. Notably missing from the list is walking, even though it is consistently identified as the most popular way to be active. It's time to get creative, break out of steady-pace walking, and design walking workouts that are fun and challenging. In this chapter, you'll learn how to take the "just" out of "just walking" and discover how to bring energy, originality, and a sense of play to what is usually considered a pedestrian activity.

Walking workouts can be as infinite as your imagination, and they'll be much more successful if they're based on the principles of physical fitness training. One of the reasons Michele wrote her first walking book, *Walk Off Weight*, was because she heard so many complaints from walkers who said they weren't getting the results that they wanted despite walking regularly. Why? Many of them were ignoring the principle of overload—the body needs a challenge to create change. The status quo—which many walking programs and groups offer—doesn't cut it. While there has been a lot of creativity, like walking challenges, and technology, such as apps and activity monitors, to motivate people to walk, there hasn't been as much programming around the principles of training that enhance results—until now.

In this chapter, we will review these principles of training and how they can be applied to walking workout classes. From there, we will review the specifics of the conditioning segment of walking workouts to encourage good walking form and increase cardio exertion. And finally, the fun stuff: We will give you a variety of drills, including steady-state (SS) conditioning, high-intensity interval training (HIIT), variable-intensity interval training (VIIT), and high-volume intensity training (HVIT) so you can design your own awesome workouts. Having a structure from which to build your walking workout classes will enhance your professionalism, make your classes more desirable, and provide greater results for your clients.

Walking Club

Case Study

Anyone can start a walking group. The Toronto Power Walkers (TPW) club was founded by a group of professional working women who started walking races and wanted more social support in their pursuit of walking fitness. In 2018, they celebrated 10 years of walking and friendship. The group has grown to about 40 members and welcomes competitive and noncompetitive walkers. All pay a nominal annual fee of $50 to cover expenses, including food at events, training, and resources such as books.

Members can participate in three group training sessions a week. Tuesday evening interval workouts are walked around a fixed-distance loop, so the group stays together. Thursday and Saturday morning walks are distance-based: short-distance explorative and long-distance race prep, respectively. Everyone knows the start and end point, usually at a restaurant or café, where people can meet after everyone finishes since they go at different speeds. Weekly emails detail the workouts, including locations and walk goals, since there is no coach leading the sessions. A weekly blog keeps the group enthused and motivated. At times, the group will hire a certified fitness trainer or coach for special workshops and guidance.

They hold quarterly meetings, and a few key members are responsible for the blog, finances, communication, and research on races and walking vacations. At their January meeting, members bring walking apparel and gear that they no longer use to share, especially for those new to the group. Anything unclaimed is donated to a local shelter.

Annually, the group leaves their walking clothes and shoes at home and gathers for a formal end-of-the-year dinner meeting. They show off the medals they won over the past year. They select charities to donate any unused funds from the annual membership fees. They plan social events and formal training for the upcoming year as well as potential races or walking vacations. In the new year, smaller groups will organize plans for the races, vacations, and training to ensure that the dreams become reality. It's a model that has worked for a decade, and they hope it will continue for many more.

Principles of Physical Fitness

General program planning and each walking class should be based on recognized fitness training principles that apply to everyone, from beginners to elite athletes. The next sections will explore how to use these principles within your walking programs.

Principle of Individual Differences

Everyone is unique. Even if two people follow the same walking program, results are likely to be different based on genetics, experiences, body shape and size, daily habits, gender, chronic conditions, and injuries. This is why it is important to get to know your clients and customize the workout for their individual needs. We'll delve more into this topic in chapter 9.

Principle of Overload

When it comes to getting results, overload is the game-changer. Just about everyone is motivated to stick with a program when they see improvements—feeling happier, sleeping better, wearing smaller sizes, or having fewer aches and pain. People come to you for training because they want to get healthier and more fit. But those improvements are only possible if walking workouts adhere to the principle of overload. That means providing a stimulus, load, or stress (in the good sense) to the body that is beyond what it is used to doing.

Principle of Adaptation

It's not enough to just overload the body. Another guiding principle of the human ability to improve is the general adaptation syndrome (GAS). After overload, positive adaptation occurs only as long as the body has appropriate time for rest and recovery.

As a coach, it's your responsibility to create appropriate challenges (or overload) while respecting the need for rest and recovery. Design fitness walking programs and classes that push your clients to a level of effort that increases heart rate, breathlessness, and sweating, and then allows them to recover from the effort. When you achieve this balance in both programs and classes, your participants will experience success, and you will leave them wanting more.

Over time, the body becomes accustomed to the overload, and improvements wane. This is commonly referred to as a plateau, and it's a point where a greater overload (principle of overload), with appropriate recovery, is needed to continue to improve.

Principle of Progression

This principle relates to the systematic process of applying overload. Too much too soon can result in injury or muscle damage. But too little can result in frustration when participants do not see improvement. A gradual increase in the workload, combined with adequate rest and recovery, is desirable for optimal gains with minimal injury risk.

Principle of Specificity

The body needs to train for the specific results desired. For instance, if a client wants to walk a marathon, doing only short interval walks won't get them to the finish line. To improve endurance for a marathon, long walks must be included in the training. Likewise, if a client wants to complete a typical four-mile walk more quickly to have more time with family, speed training is a must.

FITT Principle

This principle or guideline, which stands for frequency, intensity, time, and type (FITT) can be used to ensure that you are incorporating all the other principles into your programs and classes.

- *Frequency* refers to the number of times that the workout happens each week, for example, two or three days a week.
- *Intensity* refers to how high the heart rate or RPE gets, such as a somewhat hard effort (see table 3.1).
- *Time* means the length of each workout, such as 30 to 60 minutes.
- *Type* means the kind of movement that constitutes the conditioning aspect of the workout, for example, interval walking or strength training.

Most health and fitness organizations have published exercise recommendations based on the FITT principle that you can use as guidelines. Just remember that these are public health recommendations, meaning they are generalized for the masses. As a coach, you'll want to take them a step further and customize them to the individual needs of your clients. Most recognized health organizations currently recommend moderate to vigorous activity 5 times a week at 30 minutes per day for a total of 150 minutes a week. This is a minimum.

- The American College of Sports Medicine (ACSM) recommends exercising 3 to 5 times a week (frequency) at an intensity that is 60 to 85 percent of maximum heart rate (intensity) for 20 to 60 minutes for a total of 150 minutes (time). For strength training, they recommend doing two or three workouts a week (frequency) that target all the major muscle groups (type). One to three sets of a minimum of 8 to 10 repetitions should be done for each exercise with a weight or load that is 70 to 85 percent of a one repetition max (intensity), meaning the amount that would be possible if just one repetition were done.
- The American Heart Association (AHA) recommends 30 minutes (time) of moderate intensity (intensity) aerobic activity (type) at least

5 times per week (frequency) for a total of 150 minutes. Alternately, if you're doing vigorous (intensity) aerobic exercise (type), 25 minutes (time) at least 3 times a week (frequency) for a total of 75 minutes is recommended. In addition, moderate- to high-intensity (intensity) strengthening exercises (type) should be done at least twice a week (frequency) for additional health benefits.

Periodization

This isn't a principle, but it is a tool that can help you systematically design programs for your clients. Periodization has its roots in the theory of GAS, which describes the stages of response to any kind of stress, including exercise: shock of the stress (or overload), adaptation or resistance to the stress, and finally exhaustion that can result in injury or a decline in performance unless adequate rest and recovery occur. Periodization structures training in a way that balances stress or overload with recovery. While most research on periodization relates to its use in resistance training programs, it is also an effective tool for cardio workouts and is regularly used by endurance athletes. If you are training clients to walk half or full marathons or other race distances, you may want to explore periodization further. Here, we are going to give a basic overview that you can use to structure programs for the widest audience.

This training model organizes programs into periods that vary in intensity—mixing up hard, moderate, and easy workouts—to prevent overtraining and maximize benefits and performance. The different periods are called cycles: macrocycles, mesocycles, and microcycles.

- The microcycle is usually seven days. It is the building block that is repeated to create a mesocycle.
- The mesocycle can be anywhere from two to six weeks and is made up of microcycles. The length of a mesocycle is often four to six weeks because this is the accepted length of time needed for the human body to adapt with physiological improvements, after which it is ready for a new challenge.
- The macrocycle is usually based on a goal or plan for six months to one year that leads to a specific event.

Though we have given lengths for cycles in the list, there are no standards for the length of each cycle. Use the more traditional model of a seven-day microcycle when giving clients a structured workout prescription that they are following on days when they are not with you in class or if they are training for a specific walking event.

Clients rarely sign on for a full year or even six months of classes at a time, so you may adjust this model. Program design, after all, is as much art as science. For a walking class, it may be realistic to consider that the

Class Length

Coaching Tip

Most fitness classes are one hour. This works well in the busy schedules of most people and is suitable for most levels of fitness. Shorter classes may be necessary if you are offering onsite lunchtime workouts at the workplace or workouts for parents while their kids participate in sports practices or arts programs. And don't rule out longer sessions. Over the years, Lee has mostly offered 90-minute classes. The extra time means that the class can move farther away from the meeting place, allowing for greater variety in terms of location. You'll need to consider your audience when determining the length of your classes.

macrocycle is one six- to eight-week session of walking classes with a goal of improving the time it takes your clients to walk one mile. The mesocycle would be the class scheduling throughout the week. For example, Lee has found many people enjoy attending three classes each week, so she offers two 90-minute classes and one 60-minute class each week. Each class is separated by one day so that there is recovery time between workouts. The microcycle becomes each class designed to incorporate stress and recovery principles in a way that serves the population attending class. Typically, this means building the conditioning segment in an arc, with the first one-third dedicated to intervals or SS walking at moderate-to-high intensity effort, peaks for a third or less time at vigorous, high intensity effort, and returns to moderate-to-high intensity to finish the final third.

Parts of a Walking Workout

Each workout should consist of three important components: a warm-up, conditioning, and a cool-down. Research supports warming up muscles for 5 to 10 minutes at the beginning of a workout. The function of the warm-up is to avoid injury. It should include large body movements to promote blood flow, and warming of the muscles and tissues to prepare the body for more vigorous activity. Ideally, these body movements also mimic and target the muscles that will be used for the activity which is to follow. For example, if the warm-up is preparing for an aerobics class, there will be movement in all planes: forward and back, side to side, rotational, and up and down. See chapter 6 for a good example of a dynamic warm-up for a walking workout.

For the conditioning segment, research supports SS training, HIIT, and other interval training protocols, as well as recovery and rest to build fitness.

Get Up! Stand Up!

Research shows that all these recommendations for activity will not counteract the ill effects of sitting for eight hours. Although specific recommendations for breaking up time spent sitting is controversial, it is recommended that sitting be interspersed with standing for at least a few minutes every 60 minutes.

You may want to add a strength training component to create a circuit class and add variety to the workouts. As mentioned, the conditioning segment can be treated as a microcycle, with an arc that builds to a peak vigorous effort drill and then brings the effort level back down so that there is a seamless movement from the warm-up to the cool-down. This conditioning segment is where you combine your knowledge of physical fitness principles with your creativity and motivational skills to inspire and challenge participants to greater health and fitness. It's also where the fun and the magic happen in class. We offer conditioning workouts in this chapter so that you have tools with which to start filling your coach toolbox.

A cool-down segment could include stretching exercises. We suggest strolling for five minutes to allow the heart rate to slow down gradually. If participants were to simply come to a stop to stretch, they might experience blood pooling in the lower legs and feet. This happens when the high heart rate of the conditioning segment continues to pump blood down to those muscles of the lower body, but those muscles, no longer working at that conditioning segment effort, do not contract sufficiently to return that blood to the heart and brain. Participants might become lightheaded and may faint. Once the heart rate has diminished after the cool-down strolling, take 5 to 10 minutes to stretch while muscles, tendons, and ligaments are still warm. Use stretches from chapter 6 to improve range of motion around key joints and ultimately improve walking performance.

Now, let's take a closer look at the conditioning options that can be incorporated into workout design—the heart (so to speak) of any workout.

Conditioning

The goal of the conditioning segment is to challenge the body by encouraging physical exertion. This can be done through a range of cardiorespiratory intensities, in a limitless number of ways, in all manner of activities. This physical exertion can be maintained at an aerobic steady state, or it can vary throughout the conditioning segment in a series of intervals.

This is your opportunity to be creative and inspirational with your coaching while respecting the principles of physical activity. Watch your participants. Make sure that they are recovering between intervals in class. Ask for feedback. If you hear complaints of injury, especially injury that is not healing, revisit your approach and be prepared to recommend that a participant consider the possibility they may need more rest and recovery or assistance from a health professional. Even though walking is a low-impact, low-risk activity, injuries are still possible, especially as the intensity increases.

As a coach, you also need to consider the goals of your clients and balance the effort with enjoyment. For the very sedentary, simply getting up and walking for an hour or so several times a week, without pushing themselves to go faster, will be enough of a stress to start to deliver benefits. If they are able to talk to fellow walkers along the way, they will be more likely to come back. The first priority is always to show up. If, after a while, the consistency of the steady pace results in a fitness or speed plateau, they risk losing a sense of accomplishment. That's when you can start to push them a little harder. Some people expect you to push them right away. Get to know your clients and their goals so you can encourage the right amount of stress to give them results without discouraging them or burning them out.

Steady-State (SS) Aerobic Exertion

This consists of maintaining a consistent intensity level (as determined by heart rate or RPE) for the entire conditioning segment. There is little or no variation in intensity after the warm-up is over and before the cool-down begins. A walking class could be designed as an SS workout, although it is our experience that participants enjoy variety in their classes. If you only offer an unchanged 3K walking route each week, participants are unlikely to return. They will get bored and will not see improvement because they are not being sufficiently challenged. Still, SS exertion has a role in both maintaining and improving fitness. Many people find it easier to complete an SS walk versus a HIIT walk when walking on their own. For this reason, we recommend suggesting SS walks as a way for people to maintain fitness levels between classes.

If you want to keep participants engaged and returning to your classes, interval training provides a great tool to offer fun and variety in every class you lead. Also, interval design can be modified easily to suit individual needs. Let's take a closer look at the research that has resulted in a dramatic shift in fitness classes to include interval training.

Interval Training

Over the past decade, emerging research has exploded, identifying the efficacy of HIIT—alternating short vigorous effort bouts of activity with usually longer recovery intervals. This type of training has been used by runners since the early 1900s [1], and is credited with many world-record performances, most notably when British runner Roger Bannister became the first man to run a mile in less than four minutes in 1954 [2]. Around 50 years later, the work of several researchers, including Izumi Tabata of Japan, Martin Gibala of Canada, Jorge Zuniga of the United States, and Niels Vollaard of Scotland discovered that HIIT also accrues benefits for people simply seeking to maintain or improve fitness levels as they age. Research has shown that HIIT causes improvements to cardiorespiratory fitness similar to that of SS exercise—but in less time. That is a big plus when one of the most common excuses for not exercising is "I don't have time." And that's not the only benefit.

HIIT has been shown to be one of the most effective ways for the body to manufacture new mitochondria—the powerhouse of each body cell. Previously it was thought new mitochondria could be created in the body only through SS aerobic or endurance training. Mitochondria exist to turn the body's source of energy (carbohydrates) into its energy currency—adenosine triphosphate (ATP). Carbohydrates are to the body what coal or nuclear power is to the home. We do not operate lights, computers, and

What Does the Research Into Interval Training Mean to Us as Coaches?

HIIT versus VIIT versus HVIT? If it all seems a bit confusing, you're not alone. There is a certain level of confusion among fitness professionals around the differences and which acronym to use. For clients, calling interval training HIIT seems to resonate with what they are reading in consumer publications, even though the reality is that the intervals they perform in classes do not align perfectly with the HIIT protocols that have been tracked in a research environment. The intensity intervals they are doing in class may vary in intensity and duration and, similarly, the recovery intervals may vary in length. While researchers continue to investigate the optimal ratios of intensity, time, and recovery, fitness professionals and coaches working with the general population can be confident that a variety of intensity interval strategies will improve health and fitness for their clients. Importantly, it gives coaches the confidence to create classes that offer a limitless opportunity for drill creativity. Research even supports using interval training for such special populations as people with diabetes [3], metabolic syndrome [4], and obesity [5].

television by burning coal or plutonium in home furnaces. Coal or plutonium combustion happens at a distant generator that feeds an electrical grid. Then, we flick a switch in our homes so electricity can turn on the devices we want to use.

Food is analogous to coal or plutonium. The carbohydrates we eat are stored as glycogen in the muscles and liver. When muscle contraction is required, mitochondria convert the glycogen into ATP in the same way the generators at a power station turn coal or plutonium into electricity. If interval training increases the number of mitochondria in the body, more ATP is available to fuel muscle contraction. These new mitochondria will access and burn off stored carbohydrates even at rest. The result is increased resting metabolic rate, which means the body burns more calories at rest.

HIIT also results in the development of more capillaries. These are the smallest blood vessels in the body, where oxygen exchange happens. More capillaries in the muscle fibers allow for more efficient oxygen delivery to burn off the body's fuel, allowing for greater muscle contraction. Think of a car: Fuel is required to turn the engine on and to move forward. Fuel needs an oxygen supply to facilitate fuel combustion. Think of muscles as the engine. For the body to move forward, those muscles need fuel. In the human body, that fuel is stored carbohydrates or glycogen. To access glycogen, after its conversion to ATP in the mitochondria, it must combust with oxygen to power muscles. If more capillaries deliver more oxygen, there will be better combustion. The result is a more powerful personal engine!

All these benefits have resulted in an incredible rise in the popularity of fitness programs that include HIIT. This interest in the benefits of HIIT has led to increased research into variations of interval training, including VIIT and HVIT. We'll look at each of them and follow up with ideas for walking class design to incorporate them.

In terms of the "frequency" and "time" of the FITT principle, there is conflicting advice on protocols for these types of workouts, and more research is needed. Researchers studying intensity intervals suggest doing three or four interval workouts a week with as little as four minutes of total high-intensity intervals per session to achieve physiological improvements and meet current exercise recommendations.

You can use different intensity intervals to improve the fitness of participants while increasing the variety and fun of your workouts. It helps to understand these different types of intensity intervals and the reasons for using them.

High-Intensity Interval Training (HIIT)

This workout typically involves brief, but vigorous, bouts of exercise alternating with periods of recovery. Both the intense work phase (WP) and the recovery phase (RP) are timed. There are several protocols of HIIT training in which the length of time dedicated to intense effort remains constant and is alternated with constant lengths of recovery. Virtually all these protocols call for vigorous effort during the WP intervals, as measured by heart rate, RPE, or oxygen uptake. Studies have shown that HIIT induces positive adaptations to cardiorespiratory and bone-muscle function that is equivalent to that resulting from traditional endurance training [6].

Ongoing research on interval training continues to show its high efficacy in comparison to continuous exercise. If time is a factor in helping people get fit or reach performance expectations, interval training is the way to go. Interval training may consist of sprint interval training (all-out or maximal effort) and HIIT (vigorous, submaximal effort). Popular protocols include Tabata training, a form of interval training in which participants are led through 20-second bursts of high-intensity anaerobic movement followed by 10-second RPs repeated through 8 cycles, and the Wingate test in which participants give all-out effort for 30 seconds and then recover for 4 minutes. These protocols each consist of work interval phases performed at vigorous effort repeated for the same time duration, alternating with active RPs that are also identical in time to each other.

Encouraging such intense effort can be challenging for a walking coach. We give tips on how to do that in the drill suggestions that follow. Also, the extreme protocols of something like Tabata can be discouraging for people new to physical activity. If you offer it, keep it short and find your most empowering coaching voice to deliver it!

Variable-Intensity Interval Training (VIIT)

This type of workout is similar to HIIT except that, as the word *variable* suggests, the intensity of the intervals varies as does the timing of those intervals and the recovery intervals. These intervals can be used successfully in walking class because the intensity can be varied according to participant fitness, weather conditions, and venue opportunity or restriction. Also, you can discover your coaching creativity in many ways using VIIT. Some research supports physical fitness improvement with "non-all-out" intensity interval training that could be categorized under VIIT. You'll see a range of examples of VIIT later in this chapter.

High-Volume Interval Training (HVIT)

High-volume interval training features long work intervals, up to three to four minutes, with effort levels of 75 percent or less and RPs that are typically shorter than the high-intensity WP. Consistency of effort and duration is in the work and recovery phases. Some believe the short RP puts people at risk for injury, particularly deconditioned individuals. We have used this strategy in walking workouts but with a slight change; we make the recovery intervals equal to or longer than the high-intensity WP.

Combo of HIIT With SS

Researchers are now looking into combining HIIT with SS. This could certainly be used in a walking workout class. For example, perhaps a class has a 30-minute cardio conditioning segment. Fifteen minutes could be designated to do HIIT intervals, and the final 15 minutes could be used for SS. Or, for a 60-minute walking workout with a 40-minute conditioning segment, you can dedicate the first 20 minutes to interval training and follow that with 20 minutes of SS walking to return to your starting point. Conversely, you could begin with 20 minutes of steady pace; this is particularly helpful on cold days to ensure participants are sufficiently warmed up before beginning 20 minutes of high-intensity speed walking. Alternatively, bookend intervals of 10 minutes SS before and after the 20 minutes of high-intensity intervals.

Creating Your Walking Workouts

You are in a position to effect great change. If you challenge the people in your classes, and if you offer appropriate rest and recovery within the class and between classes, their bodies will respond by getting stronger, faster, and fitter. If you do nothing else but change up the workout every week, always ensuring that they are working to maximum capacity for at least 10 minutes of the class, clients who attend consistently will get faster and fitter. Besides being based on tested physiological principles, the variation in workouts maintains participant interest and engagement. Just as gym clients return every week to their favorite indoor cardio classes, walkers will return to your outdoor walking workout.

People often find it difficult to get out for a walk on their own. If they do, they tend to walk at a steady pace because it is easy. They leave the house, stroll to warm up, and then, hopefully, pick up the pace to get a little breathless and a little sweaty. When with a friend, a walker may pick up the pace to match that of the friend or may just as easily slow down to chat. It is ideal to get their heart rates at least into the lower target heart rate zone for a moderate cardiorespiratory workout. There is science to support that this maintains or improves health as the Physical Activity Guidelines mentioned earlier in the chapter reveal.

The interval workout is one that people are unlikely to do on their own; the effort levels may seem daunting, or individuals are often unsure if they are doing it correctly. From a coaching perspective, intensity intervals allow you to create fun classes. Yes, you could design your classes to follow strict lab-researched HIIT protocols, and for competitive athletes intent on shaving seconds off race times, that may be a good idea. But you will most likely be drawing from an inactive to somewhat active population—people whose goal is to be more physically active in an effort to be healthier and fitter. Completing a race 20 seconds faster than a previous race may end up being a goal, but on a daily basis, your participants want a fun class that makes them feel successful and invigorated.

Learn to Loop

The key to success with these walking workouts is to coach everyone in the class for the entire class, even if the paces of your participants vary significantly. The group must stay together. This requires good drill and participant management. We have had great success using a looping technique. Almost every class will include participants who walk at varying speeds and potentially people who need accommodation. The looping technique is the best way to keep the class moving together while allowing all participants to get the workout they need. Even as you begin the strolling warm-up, people will start to spread out. This will be even more true once you begin speed drills. An easy way to loop your group is to allow them to spread out during speed intervals and then have them loop back during recovery intervals. For effective leadership and safety, keep the group within earshot so that everyone can hear your instructions.

When the class starts to spread out and you feel the spread is getting too great to manage (this can happen at any time), call "Loop!" Faster walkers in the lead turn back, keeping pace, and find a place toward the back of the group. Slower walkers who were walking closer to the back of the group can keep walking without looping.

As the coach, you should stay at the back of the group once you've taught them how to do this so you can monitor everyone for safety. (For the first few minutes of class, you may need to be in the front and demonstrate how looping works.) As the faster walkers loop, encourage them to return to you so that you get a chance to chat with them. We have found that many fast walkers prefer to loop only partway back to avoid having to weave their way through slower walkers, but they are close enough to hear instructions.

Instead of vocally calling "loop," consider using a whistle. We blow three short, quick blasts of the whistle as the nonverbal cue for looping. A second set of three short, quick blasts means that everyone should return to the coach. (We use one short blast to signal the start of a speed interval and two short blasts to signal recovery.)

Looping serves several purposes. It gives the coach a chance to talk and walk with each person. Each person in the class has a chance to get to know everyone else, and it allows everyone the opportunity to work on drills together while ensuring that each participant is working at their desired pace. It allows you to offer classes to people from a range of paces, demographics, and special populations.

Periodization in classes may be helpful. Macrocycles and mesocycles can be used for annual program planning, especially if you have participants who enjoy training for races. Six- to eight-week program organization can be considered mesocycles within the macrocycle of a year. The workouts done in one week are considered microcycles.

> **Go Fast!**
>
> **Coaching Tip**
>
> Using this cue in an introductory class works well. It saves you a long discussion defining RPE. Pacing is a developed skill, and most people in an intro walk class are unlikely to push themselves so fast that they would hurt themselves.

Or, you could consider one six- to eight-week session of classes as a macrocycle. In the first class, you could choose a set distance to time participants in a benchmark walk. The weekly walking workout program would support the goal to improve the time it takes to walk that distance by the last class. Each class becomes a microcycle. Helping your participants set these types of goals can be fun and rewarding.

During classes, introduce intervals of high-intensity speed walking, alternating with recovery intervals. Please note the term *recovery*—not *rest*. Remind your students of this too! All the science research on HIIT, VIIT, and HVIT include active RPs. Active recovery in a walking class is walking, or strolling, at a pace that allows the RPE to lower from that of the WP, allowing the participant to push through the next WP.

Walking Drills

Using the guiding principles of fitness we have reviewed, you can bring variety, challenge, and fun to every conditioning segment of every walking class. Each class can be different.

If you offer walking classes that continue throughout the year, your priority may be to simply offer a variety of drills in each class so that participants stay interested and engaged. If you take a break between class sessions, consider periodizing the workouts, as mentioned earlier, so you are building to an annual or biannual benchmark. You may want to adjust the conditioning workout to allow for seasonal change. In Toronto, where Lee leads classes throughout the year, she moves the workouts to cooler trail and ravine settings in summer. The terrain necessitates a change in speed because trail walking tends to be slower than walking on asphalt roads and trails or concrete sidewalks. The heat may dictate the intensity of the drills as well. Heat stroke and dehydration need to be avoided. In winter, many roads and sidewalks become difficult to navigate. Creativity is required to use small areas that have been cleared of ice and snow.

Without the benefit of heart rate monitors or $\dot{V}O_2$max measuring equipment, how do we encourage participants to push the WP intervals to a threshold that gives them similar benefits to what has been found in research labs? When you ask participants to go as fast as possible, they often hold back a little. The mind plays a powerful role controlling the effort of muscles. Before any class begins, offering a review of what is planned during the conditioning segment is an excellent strategy to make participants comfortable and prepared. Still, when they know what's coming, their minds partition the energy available to the muscles. As a coach, we can help break through these barriers to effort.

In the drills that follow, you will notice a variety of interval training including HIIT, VIIT, and HVIT. Your audience will determine what drills you choose to use. An introductory six-week session might warrant a different approach to the mesocycles and microcycles than sessions for more experienced walkers do. An introductory session may need shorter, less-intense WP intervals and longer RP intervals. A class that has several participants training for longer walking races may benefit from longer WP intervals and equal RP. Any participants in the class not training for the race will benefit from the drill either way.

We have found that categorizing drills into two types, go-recover and self-compete, is helpful when designing the arc of the conditioning segment of class. Even after a warm-up, many participants, especially those who are new to exercise, need to build to a peak effort. Organizing drills to move participants from moderate-intensity effort to vigorous effort helps create a sense of accomplishment and success while minimizing the risk for injury. Go-recover drills are those in which you simply tell them to go or blow a whistle, and participants know that they should be walking as fast as they can until they hear you either say "Recover" or blow two whistles. In these go-recover drills, we estimate people will push to an RPE of about 7 or 8 out of 10, even though we suggest they strive for 7 to 9. These are good drills to do at the beginning and end of the conditioning segment because they are just slightly easier than self-compete drills.

In a self-compete drill, either distance or time is repeated, and racers are competing against themselves. For a distance self-compete drill, the goal is to decrease the time it takes to cover that distance with each repetition. For a timed self-compete drill, the goal is to walk farther each repetition. In these drills, we estimate that people will push to an RPE over 8. The effort we have witnessed in these self-compete drills tends toward maximal and constitutes the peak effort point of the conditioning segment.

Use the drills that follow on their own or in combination. Note that changing the timing of WP to RP can change a drill from HIIT to VIIT or HVIT. Also, keep in mind that our identification of a drill as HIIT, VIIT, or HVIT is offered as a guideline and depends on timing of WP to RP and the intensity that you assume you are getting out of your walkers. In the final analysis, whether a drill is HIIT, VIIT, or HVIT matters less than ensuring that people are challenging themselves to walk in the higher range of their RPE. Know your audience, and pay attention to participant response to the drills and conditions such as weather that might make one protocol better than another.

Go-Recover Drills

In these timed interval drills, tell people when to go fast and when to recover. Before beginning a series, suggest effort levels for both the WP and RP before saying, "Go." After you call "Recover," remind them to keep moving, possibly reminding them of the recovery effort level or letting them find an intuitively comfortable recovery pace. We suggest choosing basic timed intervals at the beginning of any program session and always at the beginning of classes. At the beginning of a program, it is a good way to ensure that everyone understands how the drills work. At the beginning of a class that has new or experienced walkers, it is a good way to advance from the warm-up to higher-intensity drills. It also helps to choose drills that feature RP longer than the WP. Progress to more challenging versions a few weeks into a program or at the peak of any class when you know the participants can manage the intensity and challenge. We have organized these example Go-Recover drills from less complex to more complex.

Note: We do not categorize these examples as HIIT because most people do not achieve an RPE of 8-9 when performing these drills. While the 30:20:10 drill, reserved for experienced participants, does demand RPE 10 exertion, it does not have standard WP and RP protocol of standard HIIT.

Basic Timed Intervals (VIIT)

WP<RP

Good for beginning or end of workout

Total Time

Approximately 6 to 10 minutes

- 6 to 10 repeats: 20 seconds (RPE 7-9) → 40 seconds (RPE 4-6)
- 4 to 6 repeats: 30 seconds (RPE 7-9) → 60 seconds (RPE 4-6)
- 5 to 8 repeats: 30 seconds (RPE 7-9) → 45 seconds (RPE 4-6)

WP=RP

Good for beginning or end of workout

Total Time

Approximately 6 to 10 minutes

- 9 to 15 repeats: 20 seconds (RPE 7-9) → 20 seconds (RPE 4-6)
- 6 to 10 repeats: 30 seconds (RPE 7-9) → 30 seconds (RPE 4-6)
- 4 to 7 repeats: 45 seconds (RPE 7-9) → 45 seconds (RPE 4-6)

WP>RP

Best for peak workout

Total Time

Approximately 6 to 10 minutes

- 5 to 8 repeats: 45 seconds (RPE 7-9) → 30 seconds (RPE 4-6)
- 7 to 12 repeats: 30 seconds (RPE 7-9) → 20 seconds (RPE 4-6)
- 12 to 20 repeats: 20 seconds (RPE 7-9) → 10 seconds (RPE 4-6)—extended Tabata

Suggested use: An entire conditioning segment could use just these drills. One set of WP<RP, one set of WP=RP, and one set of WP>RP. The timing of WP to RP can be increased. We have used WP intervals as long as two to four minutes, typically with equal RP or longer ones, depending upon your clients.

Slow-Build Pyramid (VIIT)

Total Time

17 minutes

- 3 repeats: 30 seconds (RPE 7-9) → 30 seconds (RPE 4-6)
- 3 repeats: 35 seconds (RPE 7-9) → 35 seconds (RPE 4-6)
- 3 repeats: 40 seconds (RPE 7-9) → 40 seconds (RPE 4-6)
- 3 repeats: 35 seconds (RPE 7-9) → 35 seconds (RPE 4-6)
- 3 repeats: 30 seconds (RPE 7-9) → 30 seconds (RPE 4-6)

Suggested use: This could be an entire conditioning segment, possibly preceded by 6 to 10 minutes of basic timed intervals with WP<RP.

Reducing Recovery Intervals (VIIT)

Total Time

8 minutes

- 1 repeat: 30 seconds (RPE 7-9) → 30 seconds (RPE 4-6)
- 1 repeat: 30 seconds (RPE 7-9) → 25 seconds (RPE 4-6)
- 1 repeat: 30 seconds (RPE 7-9) → 20 seconds (RPE 4-6)
- 1 repeat: 30 seconds (RPE 7-9) → 15 seconds (RPE 4-6)
- 1 repeat: 30 seconds (RPE 7-9) → 10 seconds (RPE 4-6)
- 1 repeat: 30 seconds (RPE 7-9) → 5 seconds (RPE 4-6)
- 1 repeat: 60 seconds (RPE 7-9) → 2 minutes, 15 seconds (RPE 4-6)

Suggested use: This is a great drill to do on a track or any other place where the group can walk in a circular motion, ideally with participants walking around the coach, who is in the center. This set-up works well in a drill such as this in which recovery times get really short, leaving no time for people to loop. Because this drill takes eight full minutes to complete, a group of people walking with varied paces can spread out if you are trying to do this on residential streets or a trail. When done on a circle, the coach can see everyone. Repeat the drill once in a clockwise direction and once in a counter-clockwise direction for a total of 16 minutes. This can constitute the peak component of the conditioning segment.

Increasing Recovery Intervals (VIIT)

Total Time

8 minutes

- 1 repeat: 30 seconds (RPE 7-9) → 35 seconds (RPE 4-6)
- 1 repeat: 30 seconds (RPE 7-9) → 40 seconds (RPE 4-6)
- 1 repeat: 30 seconds (RPE 7-9) → 45 seconds (RPE 4-6)
- 1 repeat: 30 seconds (RPE 7-9) → 50 seconds (RPE 4-6)
- 1 repeat: 30 seconds (RPE 7-9) → 55 seconds (RPE 4-6)
- 1 repeat: 30 seconds (RPE 7-9) → 75 seconds (RPE 4-6)

Suggested use: Just as with the reducing recovery intervals, this could be done on a track or location where people can walk in a circular motion (possibly around a green space in a park). Because of the longer RPs, this would also work in a linear fashion on trails or residential areas because there is enough time for people in the lead to return back to the main group, or to loop (see the Learn to Loop section in this chapter).

30-20-10 Intervals (VIIT)

Total Time

21 minutes

- 5 repeats: 30 seconds (RPE 5-6) → 20 seconds (RPE 6-8) → 10 seconds (9-10)
- 1 repeat: 2 minutes (RPE <6)
- 5 repeats: 30 seconds (RPE 5-6) → 20 seconds (RPE 6-8) → 10 seconds (9-10)
- 1 repeat: 2 minutes (RPE <6)
- 5 repeats: 30 seconds (RPE 5-6) → 20 seconds (RPE 6-8) → 10 seconds (9-10)
- 1 repeat: 2 minutes (RPE <6)

Suggested use: This triple-interval protocol is based on a 2012 study of moderately fit runners that showed greater benefits compared to SS running [7]. We've found that it's a way to get people to push themselves closer to their maximum potential. For that reason, it should be reserved for clients who have experience with pacing and intervals.

Hill Intervals (VIIT, HVIT)

Walking uphill is almost always a vigorous workout for participants. The recovery is easily incorporated returning downhill to begin another uphill interval. The downhill recovery is an excellent place to practice good walking form (see chapter 4 for details). Here are four ideas for fun interval work on hills.

WP<RP

Total Time

Approximately 15 minutes

Start from a position down the hill:

- 12 repeats: uphill 30 seconds (RPE 7+)
- Untimed return to downhill starting point with a focus on form (this often takes longer than the 30 seconds it took to go uphill)

WP=RP

Total Time

6 to 14 minutes

This works well on a long hill because participants walk up the hill for the WP and return downhill for the RP or walk from side to side on the hill. It is important to give them advance warning for an upcoming WP so that they have time to turn around to walk back uphill.

Start from a position down the hill:

- 4 to 7 repeats: 20 seconds (RPE 7-9) → 20 seconds (RPE 4-6)
- 3 to 5 repeats: 30 seconds (RPE 7-9) → 30 seconds (RPE 4-6)
- 2 to 3 repeats: 45 seconds (RPE 7-9) → 45 seconds (RPE 4-6)

Fountain Drill: WP>RP (VIIT)

Total Time

Dependent on the size of the hill.
Ideally anywhere from 5 to 20 minutes

Start at the bottom of the hill, moving the entire group up the hill at RPE 7 to 8. The coach walks slowly uphill at the very back of the group and calls or whistles at intermittent intervals, at which point the lead walker loops back to the coach. Keep calling or whistling at random times to have the new lead walker loop back to the coach. As the individual walkers reach the coach, they turn to head back uphill. At any given time, some of the group is heading uphill, some of the group is heading downhill, but overall the group is getting closer to the top of the hill. Eventually the entire group is at the top of the hill.

Suggested use: This drill works well to mix up who is leading the group, giving people who are typically slower and at the back of the group a chance to be up front. This drill can also be done on flat ground or going back down the hill.

You can direct the entire group down the hill at this point, or you can repeat this fountain drill back downhill so that there is still an uphill interval component.

Perpetual Motion Machine (VIIT)

Total Time

Dependent on the size of the hill.
Ideally anywhere from 5 to 20 minutes

Perform this drill on hills that have streetlamps or other regular indicators (e.g., barrier posts). Have participants walk up two posts, then back down one post, up two, down one until they have reached the top of the hill.

If you live in an area of rolling hills, it is a great idea to do standard timed intervals up and down hills. Use the decline recovery time as an opportunity for clients to practice good walking form.

Fartlek (VIIT, HVIT)

Total Time

As you choose

Untimed drills can be used in the class environment because the randomness "shocks" the body. Hill repeats can be a form of fartlek. Walking fast to specific destinations works. For example, walk every other city block fast. This is a handy drill to have in your coach tool box, should you forget your watch or its battery fails—which has happened to us!

Butterfly (VIIT, HVIT, SS)

Total Time

As you choose

This drill works well at a venue with a hill designated for pedestrians only and a flat straightaway at the bottom or top of that hill. Split the group in two. Everyone starts at either the bottom of the hill or the top. One group faces in the direction heading out onto the flat straightaway. The other group faces looking either up (if starting at the bottom of the hill) or down the hill (if starting from the top of the hill). Start both groups at the same time. One group walks out along the flat and the other group walks up or down the hill. After 15 seconds, blow a single whistle or call out. Everyone turns and walks in the opposite direction and past the starting point. The effect is that the people who were walking along the flat ground from the starting point now walk on the hill. The people who started on the hill portion are now walking out on the flat. Whistle when you want everyone to turn. This can be untimed. You are simply allowing the group to move out farther from the starting point, where you have been standing. We call this butterfly because the two groups are "drawing wings" on the ground as they go out and back.

Suggested use: This is a good drill when people need variation between intense and less intense because the hill section adds intensity and the flat section allows people to exert less effort. It's fun to have people high-five each other as they are walking past to bring a sense of play and camaraderie to the drill.

Sharing Energy (HIIT/VIIT/HVIT)

Name alternating class members after synergistic combinations. For example: wind and sail, flowers and sunlight, trees and leaves, hearts and stars. You will have two groups from which partners will be drawn. For example, there will be a "sail" partner and a "wind" partner. Determine a set time for the drill, perhaps 30 seconds up a hill. When the coach says to go, the partners walk together as fast as possible. At some point, one will pull ahead. The person who pulls ahead must slow down to "share" their energy with the partner, such as by using encouraging words. Both recover when the coach calls, "Recover." The drill is repeated with the same two partners. However, the slower partner gets a head start and the faster partner must draw upon the energy of the slower partner to catch up during the timed interval. After two intervals, they get a new partner from the other named group. For example, "sails" are always looking for a "wind" partner.

This drill is amazing because people are challenged and because it mixes up personalities in the group to build camaraderie. It does take coaching skill in terms of helping slower walkers to find a suitable place to position themselves and to encourage all participants to find their inner cheerleader. Give permission for slower people to take a good head start.

Self-Compete Drills

These are our favorite drills to get walkers to push to their most vigorous effort. They are organized so that participants compete against themselves either for time or distance. Your clients can do this during their own workouts if they have a watch, so you could effectively assign them as homework. In the class environment, they bring a sense of play to class that is fun as well as challenging. Participants, if they enjoy it, can choose to make it competitive among each other.

Use these drills as peak drills. They can be sandwiched between one or more go-recover drills to create a good mix of vigorous and less-intense effort.

Beat the Clock (HIIT/VIIT/HVIT)

Total Time

As you choose

Determine a set distance to be walked. Have all class participants find a starting landmark. In a confined area, have participants line up in a row, with faster walkers at the front and slower at the back. The coach stands at a finish point and starts the timer while signaling participants to go. As participants pass the coach, times are read out loud and participants are asked to remember their times. Repeat as many times as you want, encouraging them to beat the clock and beat their own time. It will be necessary to keep faster walkers moving beyond the finish line until the slowest walker has crossed. Then, everyone returns to their starting landmark to repeat. Encourage maximum effort! If times slow down but maximum effort is being used, it is helpful to remind participants they have probably worked to fatigue! This is good. Their bodies will adapt to that effort and fatigue to become stronger, faster, and fitter.

A good class can have several beat-the-clock drills at different distances. For example, identify distances that are approximately 30, 45, and 60 seconds long for the majority of the class members. Repeat each of these distances 3 to 5 times.

Sometimes, you might have space that can be circumnavigated for this drill. For example, if you walk around a small residential block or green space in a park, have participants circle this area several times to beat the clock and then have them change directions.

Totem (HIIT/VIIT/HVIT)

Total Time

As you choose

This drill is similar to beat the clock, but participants try to beat their distance, not the clock. Everyone finds a totem. This could be a leaf, stick, rock or creative combination. Find a starting landmark. The coach determines the interval time: 30, 45, 60, or 90 seconds. The amount of space you have available may dictate the length. Each participant holds a totem. The coach tells them to go. Participants walk as fast as possible. When the coach says, "Recover," participants place the totem on the ground and to the side. (Remind your walkers to bend at the knees, not at the waist, to put the totem on the ground. This could be a good opportunity to teach proper squatting technique.) They then walk back to the starting landmark, picking up a second totem on the way. The coach repeats the time interval, and participants walk faster, attempting to pass their original totem. If walkers pass the first totem (and they usually do), they leave the second totem on the ground and off to the side as a new mark to beat, taking the first totem with them. If they have not passed the first totem, they return to the start with their second totem and attempt to pass on the next interval. Doing three to five repeats is usually a good amount for any of the interval times, but you can adjust the number to best suit your participants.

The RP of these drills is untimed but is always longer than the WP. If it is hot or people seem to need more recovery time, introduce an easy stretch (possibly a back extension or twist) before setting them off on the next WP.

This drill is effective in almost any season. In good weather and when the sidewalk or road is dry, it is fun to use chalk. Have participants draw a heart or star on the pavement as a starting point. When "Recover" is called, they draw a personal totem on the pavement! We believe chalk leaves a temporary mark of inspiration to anyone who happens to walk by later—a random act of happiness. At the same time, we are mindful as coaches to leave no trace in the outdoor environment. If you live in an area where chalk would not be washed away by rain, you may want to consider simply placing stones or other natural markers at the start and finish instead of using chalk.

Counting Steps (HIIT/VIIT/HVIT)

Using standard timed drills of 30-second WP, have participants count steps. (Racewalkers will achieve approximately 100 steps in 30 seconds.) Repeat the intervals, asking participants to try to get more steps in the 30 seconds. This drill can be done in 45-second and 60-second drills, where the coach says, "Go" and then shouts, "Count" for the last 30 seconds to ensure participants are keeping a good pace.

This drill also works well using Tabata training: Have people walk as fast as they can, counting steps for 20 seconds. Recover walk for 10 seconds. Repeat through 8 cycles for a total time of 4 minutes. By counting their steps through these 20 seconds, they have a measurement that motivates them to maintain intense effort and exertion.

Suggested use: This is a good drill to encourage the short, quick steps taught as part of good walking form because that is one way walkers can increase their 30-second step count. Of course, any length of drill could be used to count steps to maintain cadence. Count steps for 15, 20, 25, or more seconds. Or ask people to walk their fastest for 60 seconds, counting the steps in the last 15 seconds only to be sure they are maintaining cadence and effort through the entire WP interval. We use this drill a lot when participants get too busy chatting with each other rather than walking fast. It is impossible to count steps and talk at the same time!

Enhancing Technique

Cueing for good walking technique during any drill can be helpful to participants. Alternatively, it can be nice to simply let people enjoy the intensity challenge in itself without excessive instruction regarding form. You can use other drills to bring awareness back to technique. These drills do not challenge cardiorespiratory fitness the same way as go-recover or self-compete drills do, so they are ideal at the beginning or end of the conditioning segment or during a time when your programming plans include workouts with less intensity.

Agility Ladder Drill

To help clients practice taking shorter steps, lay one or more agility ladders out around a track or path. The number you use and how you arrange them will depend upon how many walkers you have. As they come to the ladders, instruct them to step in between each rung. This will necessitate that they shorten their steps.

One-Leg Propulsion (VIIT)

This is a pyramid-style drill using WP time and RPE as variables. During each WP, the participant should intentionally power with one leg only, beginning on the right. Ask them to visualize that leg pulling back to power the body.

- Right leg: 3 repeats; 20 seconds (RPE 5-6) → 20 seconds (RPE 6-7) → 20 seconds (8-9)
- Repeat on the left
- Right leg: 3 repeats; 30 seconds (RPE 5-6) → 30 seconds (RPE 6-7) → 30 seconds (8-9)
- Repeat on the left

Consider this: Focusing on one-leg propulsion can make the gait feel awkward and lopsided. It helps to mention this to participants before starting the drill. Also, this is a complex drill for the brain. It can challenge participants to maintain focus on the single-leg propulsion and increase RPE. One way to make it easier is to practice the drill on a decline first. On the decline, even at quick speeds RPE may stay low. Encourage them to practice powering with one leg without going fast so that they can get the feel for how it works.

Circuit-Style Drills With Strength Exercises

The strength exercises suggested in chapter 7 could be used for a walk circuit class. You could use the same exercises for four to six weeks so that clients notice improvement in the muscles being worked. We suggest using basic timed go-recover drills to alternate with strength exercises. The variations for alternating timed intervals with strength exercises are limited only by your imagination.

Both workouts that follow use resistance bands or tubes. Unlike dumbbells, a resistance band or tube can be an ideal walking companion. Doing band exercises while walking provides additional upper-body toning and strengthening—a cardio and strength combo workout. It's also a good option when weather conditions are not conducive to pushing the intensity or speed.

Keep in mind that participants may want to wear gloves when performing strength moves that require putting their hands on the ground or outdoor equipment.

Three-Minute Interval: Two-Set Strength Circuit

- 3 repeats: 20 seconds (RPE 7-9) → 40 seconds (RPE 4-6)
- 2 sets, 12 × R, 12 × L, step-together traveling lunge (p. 113)
- 3 repeats: 20 seconds (RPE 7-9) → 40 seconds (RPE 4-6)
- 2 sets, 12 × R, 12 × L, standing leg abduction (p. 121)

- 3 repeats: 20 seconds (RPE 7-9) → 40 seconds (RPE 4-6)
- 2 sets, 12 × R, 12 × L, standing leg adduction (p. 121)
- 3 repeats: 20 seconds (RPE 7-9) → 40 seconds (RPE 4-6)
- 2 sets, 12 × basic lat pull-down (p. 124)
- 3 repeats: 20 seconds (RPE 7-9) → 40 seconds (RPE 4-6)
- 2 sets, 12 × basic push-up from elevated bench/picnic table/railing/rock (p. 131)
- 3 repeats: 20 seconds (RPE 7-9) → 40 seconds (RPE 4-6)
- 2 sets, 12 × R, 12 × L, side plank with hip drop and raise (p. 129)

A four- to six-week session doing this workout could be followed by another four- to six-week session doing the same exercises but with more challenging variations.

Walk and Tone

After warming up, alternate two- to five-minute intervals of brisk walking with intervals of the band exercises done while walking. Do 10 to 15 reps. If you want to do multiple sets of an exercise, do a shorter (1 to 2 minutes) walking interval between the sets, or do one set of each exercise and then repeat the circuit. It's natural to slow the pace when doing the band exercises. The exercises that follow can be done while walking.

- *Chest press*—Place the exercise band around the back and under the armpits. Hold an end in each hand by the shoulders, palms facing down. Extend arms straight out in front, keeping arms parallel to the ground. Hold for a second then slowly return to starting position.
- *Pull-down*—Hold a band overhead, hands about 12 to 16 inches apart. Pull hands down and out to the sides, stretching the band to about chest level. Slowly raise arms back overhead to the starting position.
- *Overhead press*—Place the exercise band around the back and under the armpits. Hold an end in each hand by the shoulders, palms facing forward. Extend arms straight up overhead. Hold for a second, then slowly return to starting position.
- *Single-arm row*—Hold a band out in front, arms parallel to the ground and hands about six inches apart. Palms should be facing each other, elbows bent slightly. Keep the left arm stationary to anchor as the right elbow bends and pull the right hand pulls back, stretching the band, toward the hip. Hold for a second. Slowly straighten the arm back to the starting position. Do all reps with right arm, then repeat with left arm.
- *Triceps press*—Rest the exercise band around the back of the neck. Hold an end in each hand by the shoulders, palms facing down and elbows pointing back. Extend the arms straight down in front, keeping the arms close to the body. Hold for a second. Slowly return to starting position.

You can also stop and do stationary band exercises, like biceps curls or lateral squats with the band tied around the calves. You can loop the band around objects like railings or poles to do leg abduction and adduction for even more variety. Be creative.

Now that you see how varied walking can be, we hope that you are excited to bring these ideas and more to your walking classes. As you do, you'll want to incorporate a dynamic warm-up and cool-down stretch to increase mobility around all the joints used when walking as well as to improve walking performance. In the next chapter, we'll discuss what to focus on during these stretches.

References

1. Billat, L.V. 2001. "Interval Training for Performance: A Scientific and Empirical Practice." *Sport Medicine* 31: 13-31.
2. Earnest, C.P. 2008. "Exercise Interval Training: An Improved Stimulus for Improving the Physiology of Prediabetes," *Medical Hypotheses* 71 (5): 752-61.
3. Jakobsen, I., Solomon, T., and Karstoft, K. 2016. "The Acute Effects of Interval-Type Exercise on Glycemic Control in Type 2 Diabetes Subjects: Importance of Interval Length. A Controlled, Counterbalanced, Crossover Study." *PLOS ONE* 11. doi: 10.1371/journal.pone.0163562.
4. Mora-Rodriguez, R., Ramirez-Jimenez, M., Fernandez-Elias, V.E., Guio de Prada, M.V., Morales-Palomo, F., Pallares, J.G., Nelson, R.K., and Ortega, J.F. 2018. "Effects of Aerobic Interval Training on Arterial Stiffness and Microvascular Function in Patients with Metabolic Syndrome." *The Journal of Clinical Hypertension* 20 (1): 11-18. doi: 10.1111/jch.13130.
5. Su, L., Fu, J., Sun, S., Zhao, G., Cheng, W., Dou, C., and Quan, M. 2019. "Effects of HIIT and MICT on Cardiovascular Risk Factors in Adults with Overweight and/or Obesity: A Meta-Analysis." *PLoS One* 14 (1): e0210644. doi: 10.1371/journal.pone.0210644.
6. Gibala, M.J. 2007. "High-Intensity Interval Training: A Time-Efficient Strategy for Health Promotion?" *Current Sports Medicine Reports* 6 (4): 211-13. https://doi.org/10.1007/s11932-007-0033-8.
7. Gunnarsson, T.P. and Bangsbo, J. 2012. "The 10-20-30 Training Concept Improves Performance and Health Profile in Moderately Trained Runners." *Journal of Applied Physiology* 113 (1): 16-24. www.physiology.org/doi/full/10.1152/japplphysiol.00334.2012.

6

Stretch for Mobility and Performance

Think about waking up in the morning and taking that first really big stretch. Ahh. We've all experienced this delicious moment. By sharing the pleasure of stretching with your classes along with the high-energy parts, you'll exceed expectations as a coach.

The Power of Stretching

It helps to understand what stretching does. Many people think of it as lengthening tightened muscles, losing sight of the fact that flexibility is about the range of motion that happens around a joint. That shift in perspective changes what stretches do and how to do them.

People may have poor flexibility at all joints or limited range of motion around one or a few. How significant that range of motion is around specific joints has something to do with genetics and a lot to do with what people do every day. If they are sitting for 12 hours a day—hips and knees bent, back flexed—range of motion around these joints is going to be extremely limited. This leads to a life of dis-ease.

For happy and functional daily living, people should be able to easily do daily tasks: stand, walk, rise from sitting, bend to pick up something from the floor, reach to get something from a high cupboard, twist to check over the shoulder while driving, and more. Some people have specific range-of-motion challenges depending on their preferred leisure activities, whether it be cycling, golf, tennis, kayaking, hiking, skiing, skating, curling, and other activities that involve repetitive motion.

Walking is a fundamental life movement, and to do it well, good range of motion at the shoulders, hips, ankles, and torso in all planes is essential. The stretches offered here are a good starting point to breathe some space into these joints. Improving range of motion at the front of the hips and shoulders improves posture and walking speed. Opening the anterior deltoid (front of shoulder) and releasing the chest muscles will allow the back muscles to pull the body into a neutral spine. Opening the anterior hip joint allows the spine to sit tall over the pelvis. Interestingly, this all has a positive effect on walking speed, even more so if the posterior range

The Anatomy of Walking

What is a neutral spine? The spine has natural curves to it. When viewing a body from the side, a neutral spine reveals those curves: lordotic (anterior) curve in cervical spine (neck), kyphotic (posterior) curve in the thoracic spine (chest and upper back), lordotic curve in the lumbar spine (lower back), and kyphotic curve in the tailbone. The best way to check your clients is to look at them from the side and see that the ears stack over the shoulders, hips, knees, and center of the foot.

of motion around the ankle is improved. Range of motion at the ankle is increased by stretching the muscles of the calf. As we discussed in chapter 5, to increase walking speed, we want the toe push to happen as far behind the body's center of gravity as possible. This requires that the front of the hip joint and the back of the ankle joint are flexible enough to allow that leg to move back. Simultaneously, the anterior shoulder and chest muscles must allow the arm to swing back in a synchronous movement with the leg. If the shoulder will not allow the arm to move back, the legs will not move back because they swing in opposition with the same timing.

The Myth of Stretching as Injury Prevention

As coaches, we often hear a client say, "I have to stretch so I don't get injured." This is most likely untrue. Reviews of the research on the effects of static stretching and risk of injury show little to no benefit [1]. Considering the common causes of injuries, it makes sense that stretching doesn't play a significant role in preventing them. Many injuries not caused by a catastrophic event like a fall tend to be caused by seemingly innocuous situations. If a person sits at a desk all day, leaning slightly toward the computer, with one leg crossed over the other, postural or muscular imbalances are pulling the body out of alignment. One side is unfavorably stressed and eventually weakens. Wearing a purse over one shoulder, day in and day out for years, can have a similar effect. These weaknesses can lead to injury. In a way, these actions are like an overuse injury. An overuse injury results from repeating the same motion, or being in the same position, day in and day out, placing a cumulative stress on a specific area of the body.

Another common path to injury is to make a sudden movement for which the muscles, tendons, and ligaments are not prepared. This can happen in everyday life: The cell phone drops from your hand, and you make a sudden movement to catch it. While you are relaxing in front of the television, a child screams from another room, so you jump up to find out what is wrong. It can happen during a walking workout if the body has been poorly warmed before fast walking or high-intensity interval drills begin.

Walk to Warm Up

Coaching Tip

Lee has walked thousands of miles training for more than 30 marathons and hundreds of shorter-distance races. Every one of her training walks, whether it be a session of 800-meter speed drills, a HIIT workout, a tempo walk, or a long-distance workout, has begun with a simple stroll for five to ten minutes before slowly increasing the pace. This is great advice for your clients for their own workouts because it removes one barrier that might stop them from going out for a walk. If they think they need to do a series of stretches, many of which they may not be able to remember on their own, they may not go out for the walk.

As a coach, it is your responsibility to manage this risk in class as best as possible. It helps to remind your clients how the body can get injured and give them tips for warm-ups that they can do when walking on their own. Unlike static stretching, where it is recommended to hold a position for 30 seconds, a dynamic warm-up appears to offer more benefits pre-workout [2]. Dynamic movements without long static stretches loosen up joints, increase range of motion, wake up the nervous system, and warm up tissues throughout the body, which helps cells get the oxygen and energy demanded by exercise. At least part, or even all, of a warm-up should mimic the movements of the activity you will be doing. For an appropriate warm-up, see Dynamic Stretches section later in this chapter.

The Group Warm-Up

In a class environment, there are people of varying paces and fitness levels, so the simplest way to begin a walking class is to walk! We recommend a strolling warm-up for 5 to 10 minutes, depending on how much time you have for the whole class, with instructions that everyone set an easy pace, arms hanging by their sides and extended at the elbows. Still, even at a stroll, people will walk at different paces. The psychological dynamics of a group means that some people feel they must walk quickly to keep up with faster walkers, while others slow down to stay with the group. A coach needs to set everyone up for success. Both situations leave your participants vulnerable to muscle strain or tears when you begin the vigorous walking drills. What you do during this strolling warm-up and in a group dynamic stretch will have everyone ready for the workout.

For the warm-up stroll, tell everyone to walk at a pace that feels comfortable to warm up their bodies. To get to know your walkers and their paces, try to connect with as many as possible during the warm-up stroll, chatting with them and helping each set a pace that is appropriate. You can tell a lot by how easy or difficult it is for people to chat with you. If you have a couple of very slow walkers in class and faster ones are getting too far ahead, get the faster ones to return to the slower walkers as part of their strolling warm-up. A good technique for keeping people together is explained in the Learn to Loop section in chapter 5.

As mentioned, simply strolling will suffice as a reasonable warm-up, especially when people are walking on their own. Typically, people will self-regulate, finding a pace that ensures they will not injure themselves before moving into faster walking and even interval speed drills. When leading a group, you can add to the structure of a class and ensure that everyone warms up properly before the cardio workout begins by offering a dynamic stretching warm-up along with a strolling warm-up. For a dynamic warm-up, introduce whole-body movements that increase the range of motion around the joints while increasing blood flow to large muscle groups, as described in the next section.

Dynamic Stretches

Find a suitable location with space for the group to gather and guide them through a series of dynamic movements that will enhance blood flow to the large muscle groups. This is also a perfect opportunity to state the plan for the workout, review any safety concerns for the day, and congratulate any members on walking achievements. Then, follow this dynamic stretch routine with a focus on opening the chest, shoulders, hips, and ankles and warming up muscles that surround those joints to have everyone in the class ready for the walking workout. Here are some general guidelines to follow in performing dynamic stretches.

- The movements are made with every breath cycle. It is only after the walking workout that stretches are held for up to 30 seconds.
- Some of these dynamic movements require balancing skills. It can be helpful to do these exercises in a location where clients can put a hand on something stable to maintain balance—a wall, railing, tree, bench, or another person. Alternatively, people can partner up to hold on to each other (placing a hand on your partner's shoulder, for example) for stability.
- For those who want to use these moves as balance exercises, cue them to find a steady focal point ahead of them, pull the navel to the spine, and squeeze the shoulder blades together and down before lifting one leg off the ground.
- This is an opportunity for the class to catch up with each other. We find that people often talk among themselves. It is a perfect time for the coach to ask questions. A simple "How are you doing?" often brings out meaningful responses and helps you understand where participants are psychologically and physically.
- Keep it fun and light!

Mall Walking

Case Study

The Virginia Hospital Center was on to something when it started its free Walk-Fit mall walking program more than 20 years ago. Since it began, every Tuesday and Thursday morning, staff from the health promotion department of the hospital greet anywhere from 15 to 30 people who are willing to face rush-hour traffic and commutes of up to 45 minutes to arrive at the Fashion Centre in Pentagon City to walk laps around the mall.

Mall walking programs are good options in areas where walking outdoors may not be safe due to infrastructure, traffic, or weather. Many malls open before stores do and allow community members to walk the hallways. The controlled climate, level walking surfaces, and security make it a welcoming environment, especially for older adults, those with mobility issues, or those who use assistive walking devices. The hallways are usually wide and free of obstacles, and amenities like accessible restrooms, benches to rest on, water fountains, good lighting, and music make it an even more enjoyable experience. And seeing the same faces every morning creates a community that motivates people to keep coming back.

The Walk-Fit program's structure also helps to keep people coming back. Some walkers have joined via referral from a health specialist, but most have joined after learning about it from friends. Everyone receives a name tag and card to track their mileage and progress. Participants check in with hospital staff between 8:00 and 8:30 a.m. Then, a staff member leads a group stretch before everyone starts their quarter-mile loops. Afterward, that day's mileage is recorded, and a nurse measures blood pressure. Most participants wrap up by going for coffee in the food court with their fellow walkers. The social aspect is key to member retention, says Gwendolyn Beck, manager of senior health at the hospital.

For more information on mall walking, go to www.cdc.gov/prc/mall_walking.html.

ARM CIRCLES

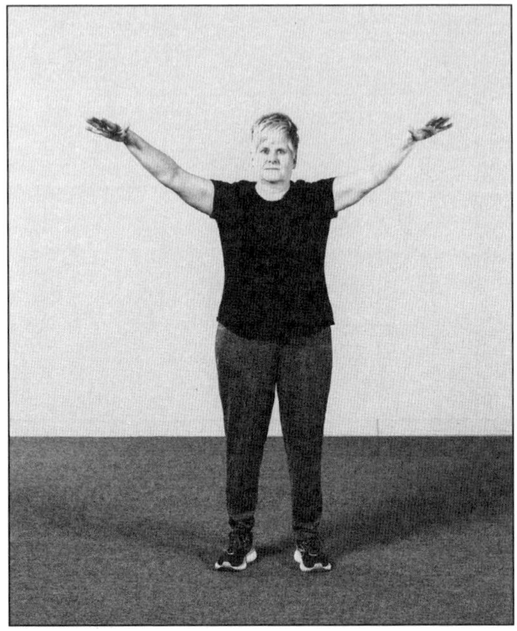

FIGURE 6.1 Arm circles.

1. Stand with the feet under the hips and arms out to the sides, palms down. Circle the arms slowly, starting with small circles and moving to larger ones, forward and then back (figure 6.1).
2. Do 8 to 12 circles in both directions.

SIDE BEND

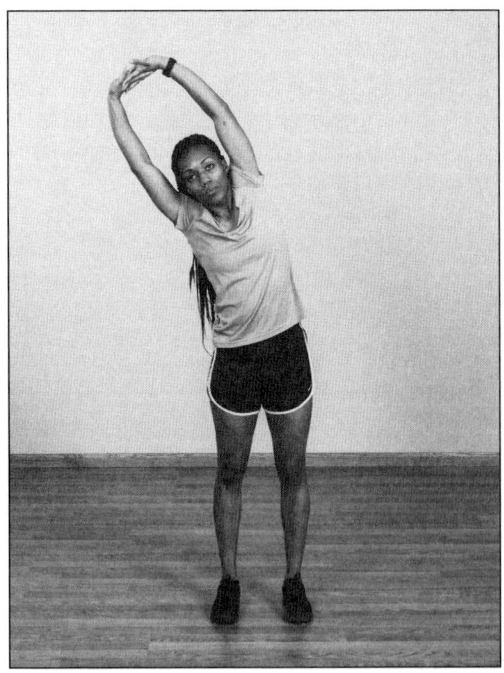

FIGURE 6.2 Side bend.

1. Inhale to bring the arms up overhead, interlace the fingers, and flip the palms toward the sky. Reach the chest forward and the hands back slightly. Maintain a neutral spine.
2. Exhale to bend at the waist, leaning to the right side as far as possible. Keep feet under hips, not letting the left hip go out to side (figure 6.2).
3. Inhale to bring the arms up overhead, then exhale to release the arms down to sides.
4. Inhale to bring the arms up overhead and interlace the fingers so the thumb on top in step 1 is now on the bottom. Flip the palms toward the sky. Reach the chest forward and the hands back slightly. Maintain a neutral spine.
5. Exhale to bend at the waist, leaning to the left side as far as possible.
6. Inhale to bring the arms up overhead, then exhale to release the arms down to the sides.

BACK EXTENSION

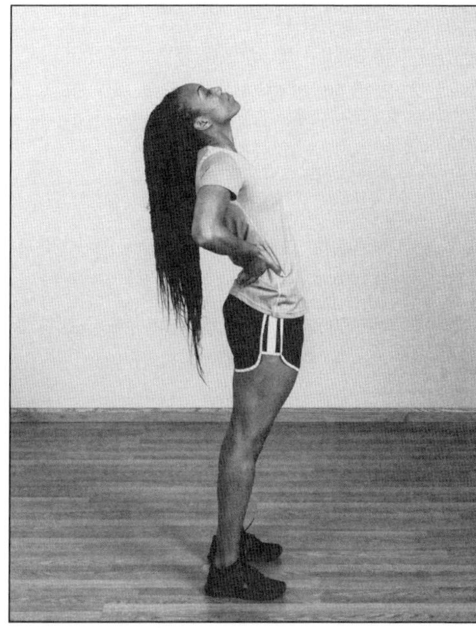

FIGURE 6.3 Back extension.

1. Inhale to place the hands in a comfortable position with the palms on the low back, simultaneously lifting the chest toward the sky and extending the spine (figure 6.3).
2. Exhale to return to standing tall, bringing the arms down to the sides. (One time only.)

TORSO TWIST

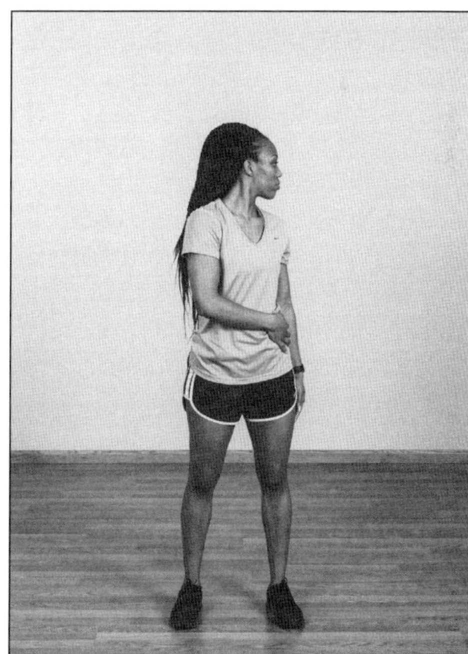

FIGURE 6.4 Torso twist.

1. Inhale to reach the right hand across the front of the body to the left hip. Let the left arm relax down to the side.
2. Exhale and use the right hand to gently twist the upper body to the left (figure 6.4).
3. Inhale to return to center.
4. Reach the left hand to the right hip; right arm relaxing down the side.
5. Exhale and use the left hand to gently twist the upper body to the right.
6. Inhale to return to center and return the arms to the sides.

LEG EXTENSION

1. Lightly hold on to a wall, railing, or tree with the right hand and shift the weight to the right leg. Inhale to bend the left hip and knee to as close to 90 degrees as possible, lifting the leg.
2. Exhale to extend the leg to straight without locking it (figure 6.5).
3. Inhale to bend the left knee back to the starting position.
4. Repeat flexion and extension at the knee 6 to 8 times.
5. Lower the foot to the ground. Switch sides and repeat steps 1 through 4 with the right leg.

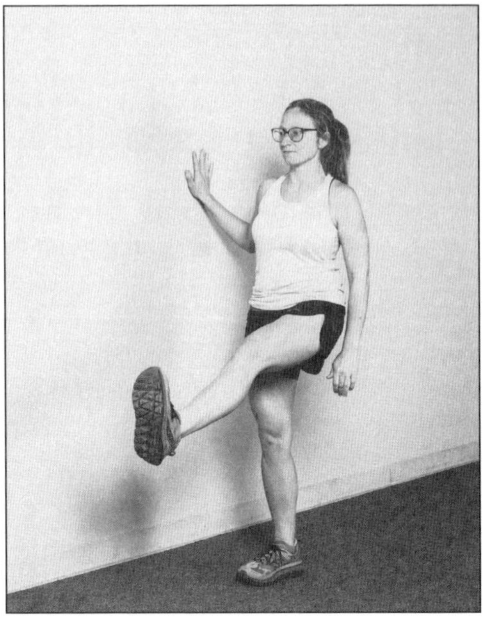

FIGURE 6.5 Leg extension.

LEG SWING

1. Lightly hold on to a wall, railing, or tree with the left hand and shift weight to the left leg.
2. Inhale and lift the right leg in front as high as possible (figure 6.6).
3. Exhale and swing the right leg back behind you, without the right foot touching the ground.
4. Do 6 to 8 leg swings on the right.
5. Repeat swinging the left leg.

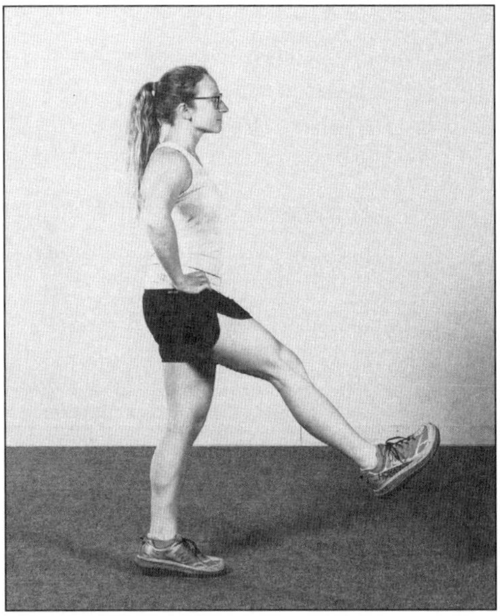

FIGURE 6.6 Leg swing.

CALF PUMP

1. Bring hands to hips and shift weight to the left leg. Step back with the right foot and bend the left knee into a slight lunge. Lightly hold on to a wall, railing, or tree if needed for balance.
2. Inhale to lift the right heel off the ground (figure 6.7a).
3. Exhale to lower the heel back down to the ground (figure 6.7b).
4. Repeat lifting and lowering the right heel for 6 to 8 times.
5. Exhale to return the right foot next to the left one.
6. Switch legs and repeat lifting and lowering the left heel.

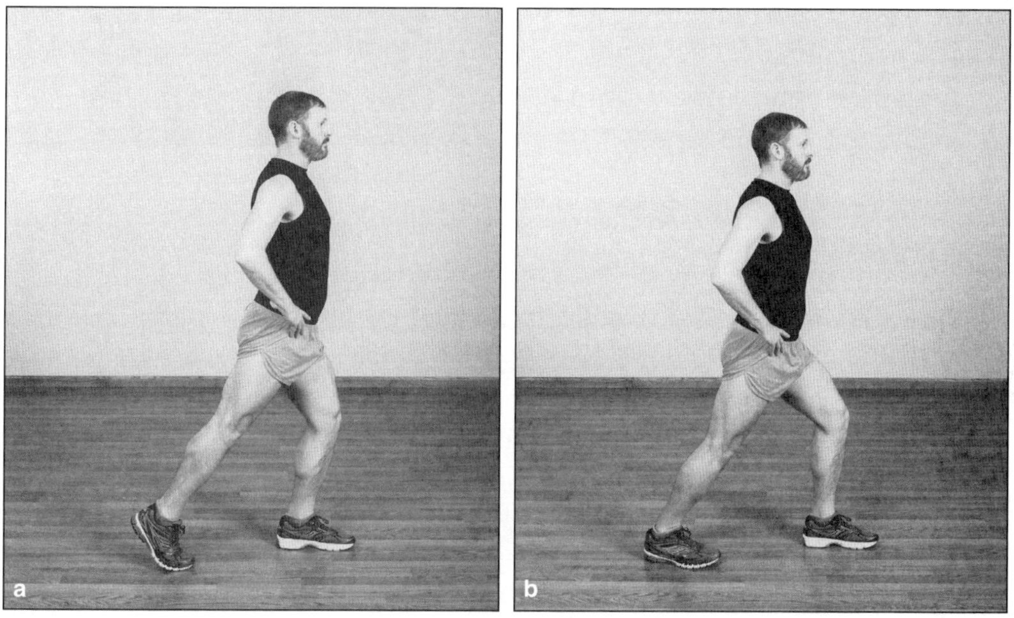

FIGURE 6.7 Calf pump.

ARM SWING

1. Bring hands to hips and shift weight to the left leg. Step back with the right foot, planting the heel into the ground.
2. Relax the arms at the sides, then swing one arm forward as the other arm swings back (as if walking) 6 to 8 times (figure 6.8).
3. Bend the arms at the elbows and continue swinging them forward and back (as if power walking) 6 to 8 times.
4. Exhale to return hands to hips, and step the right foot next to the left one.
5. Switch legs and repeat.

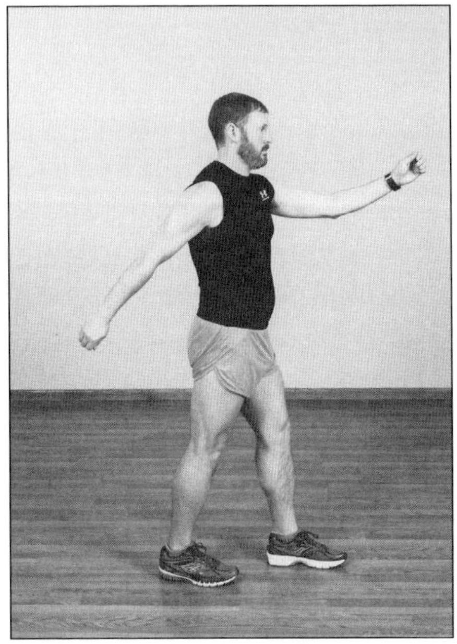

FIGURE 6.8 Arm swing.

FOOT ROLL

1. Stand with both feet directly under the hips and hands at hip level; the hands can rest on a railing or wall for stability.
2. Inhale to lift the toes and roll back onto the heels (figure 6.9a).
3. Exhale to lift heels and roll forward onto the toes and balls of feet (figure 6.9b).
4. Repeat this rolling back and forth 8 to 10 times.

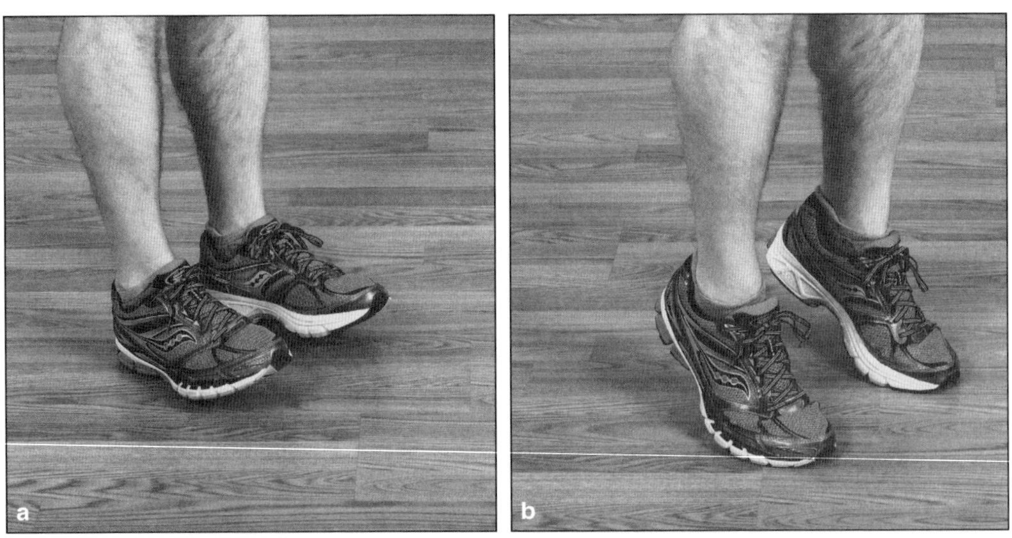

FIGURE 6.9 Foot roll.

After this dynamic warm-up, clients are ready for the cardio fun to begin. The walking workout can be designed in many ways using ideas from chapter 5. After the workout segment of class, a five-minute stroll to cool down is a natural way to transition to static stretching exercises held for a longer time that will stretch the warm muscles, tendons, and ligaments to increase flexibility.

Performance Stretches for Postworkout

These stretches are an opportunity to improve range of motion around key walking joints, especially targeting the muscles anterior to the hip and shoulder and posterior to the ankle. This can improve walking technique, speed, and overall performance.

Many factors affect the time required to see improvement from stretching. Some of these factors include age, specific muscles stretched, previous injury, hydration, fatigue level, and temperature. Still, most of the research points to considerable effectiveness from a static hold stretch of 30 seconds performed twice for a total of 60 seconds [3]. Because most people will take 8 to 10 cycles of inhalation and exhalation over 30 seconds, we recommend using breath cycle count as an effective guide for maintaining a stretch position. As your class participants count out their breath cycles in position, you may use this opportunity to give verbal cues to maximize the stretch.

Each stretch that follows should be performed twice to meet the 60-second guidelines. Joints and muscles involved in each stretch are identified, and figure 6.10 shows where to find each muscle in the body, so you can fully understand what's being stretched.

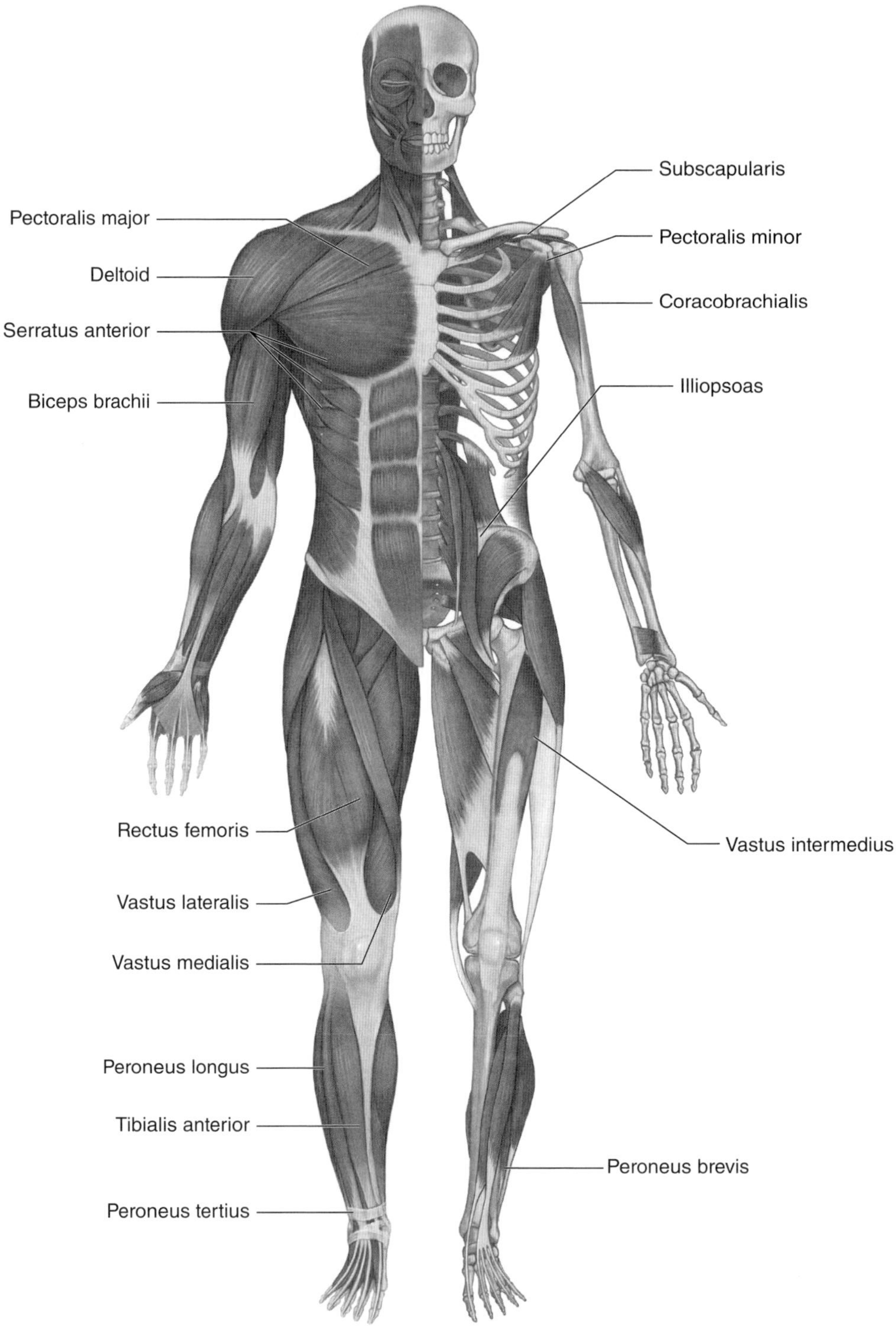

FIGURE 6.10 Human muscular system.

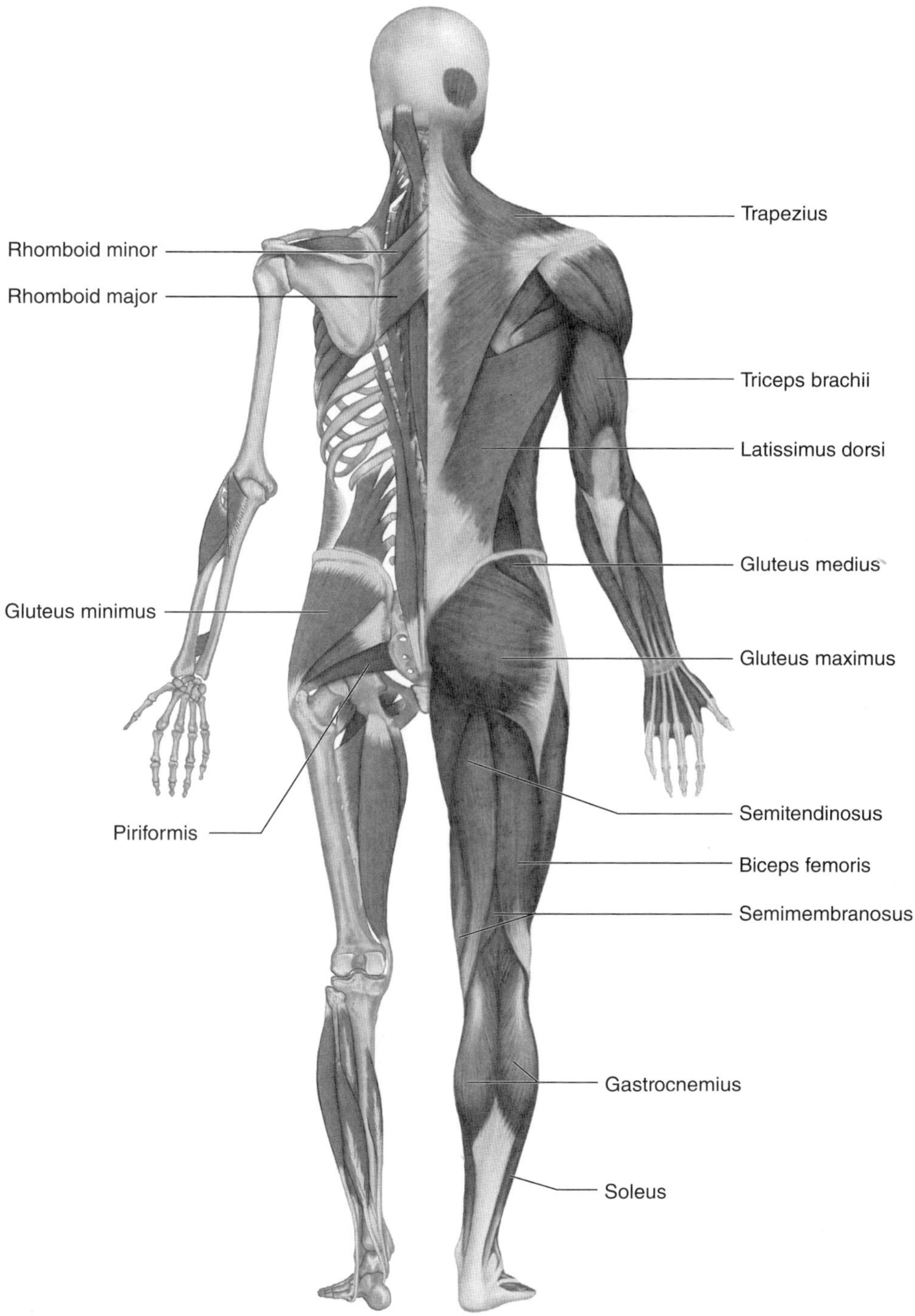

FIGURE 6.10 *(continued)*

Lower Body

CALF

Joints Targeted

Posterior ankle

Muscles Targeted

Gastrocnemius, soleus

GASTROCNEMIUS STRETCH WITH WALL

1. Stand facing a wall, the feet under the hips. Place the hands at shoulder height and width on the wall. Arms should be straight. (If a wall is not available, use a railing or tree.)
2. Inhale to step back with both feet, pressing the heels into the ground and keeping the legs straight, but not locked, through the knee joint to feel a stretch in the calf (figure 6.11).
3. Maintain position for 8 to 10 breath cycles.
4. *Optional:* For a deeper stretch, bend the elbows and move the chest closer to the wall while keeping the legs straight.
5. Exhale and step forward to starting position.

Variation

- Lift and spread the toes while holding the stretch to allow the plantar muscles, tendons, and ligaments of the foot to lengthen as well.

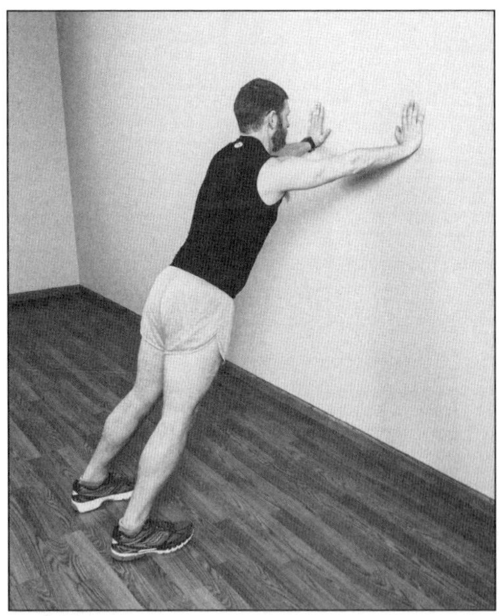

FIGURE 6.11 Gastrocnemius stretch with wall.

GASTROCNEMIUS STRETCH WITHOUT WALL

1. Stand with the feet underneath the hips and the hands at the hips.
2. Inhale to slide the right foot back slowly, maintaining the foot forward, neutral position.
3. Exhale to press the heel into the ground.
4. Inhale to bend the front left knee as necessary, keeping the spine tall and the rib cage lifted to feel the stretch through the calf (figure 6.12).
5. Maintain this position for 8 to 10 breath cycles.
6. This can be followed by 8 to 10 breath cycles, with the front knee bending a bit more and the back leg remaining in the straight-knee position to deepen the stretch.
7. Exhale and step the back foot forward to the starting position.
8. Repeat with the left leg back.

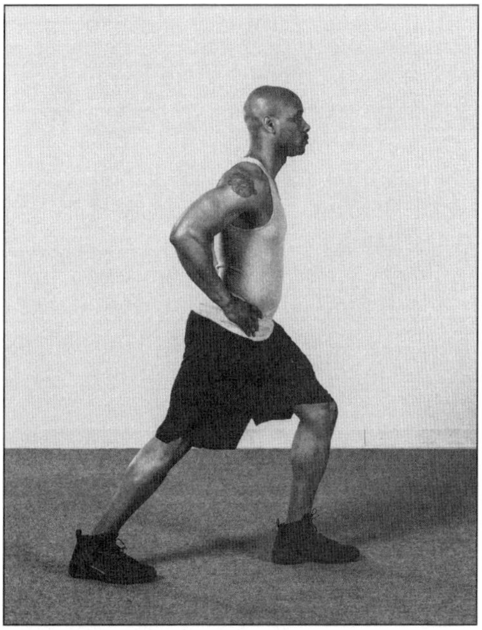

FIGURE 6.12 Gastrocnemius stretch without wall.

Variation

- Place the hands in a comfortable position on the low back and extend the back, reaching the chest toward the back, reaching the chest toward the sky, to stretch through the front of the body. Interlace the fingers behind the low back and lift the arms and hands behind to stretch the chest (figure 6.13).

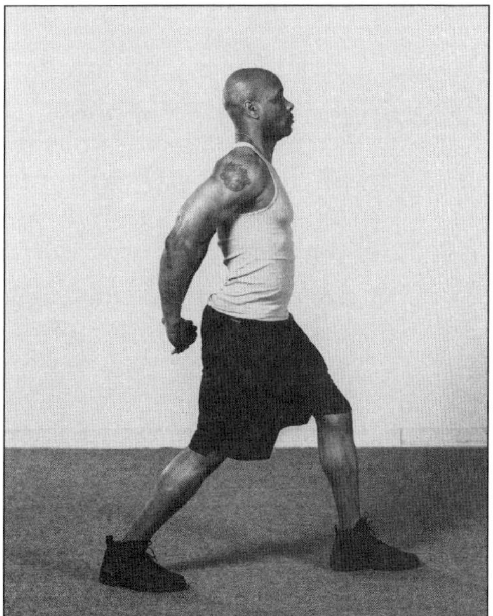

FIGURE 6.13 Gastrocnemius stretch without wall, variation.

Consider This

Using the wall (or railing or tree) for a two-leg stretch is our preferred method for gastrocnemius and soleus stretches because people tend to keep the feet pointing straight ahead, which provides stretch in the direction their feet take when walking. If no wall is available, it is important to position the back foot with the toes pointing forward. Turning them away from the midline is a common misalignment because a turned-out foot offers greater stability and allows people to step back farther, which they believe is better.

Create Body Awareness

Coaching Tip

Encourage walkers to tune in to their bodies while stretching without any judgement as to how flexible other people in the class may be. Sometimes it helps to ask them to close their eyes to bring a strong awareness to what the body is feeling rather than making a visual assessment of themselves relative to others. Help them to identify the specific areas of the body that are being stretched and ask them if they can feel it. Encourage them to let you know if they don't feel it, and remind them that everybody has a different anatomical structure. Then, guide them into a position where they do feel the stretch.

SOLEUS STRETCH WITH WALL

1. Stand facing a wall, the feet under the hips. Place the hands at shoulder height and width. The arms should be straight. (If a wall is not available, use a railing or tree.)
2. Inhale to step back with both feet.
3. Exhale to press the heels into the ground, keeping the legs straight through the knee joint, but not locked, to feel a stretch in the calf.
4. Inhale to gently bend the knees slightly, keeping the heels glued to the ground, to feel a stretch in the lower calf, closer to the Achilles tendon (figure 6.14).
5. Maintain the position for 8 to 10 breath cycles.
6. Exhale and step the back foot forward to the starting position.

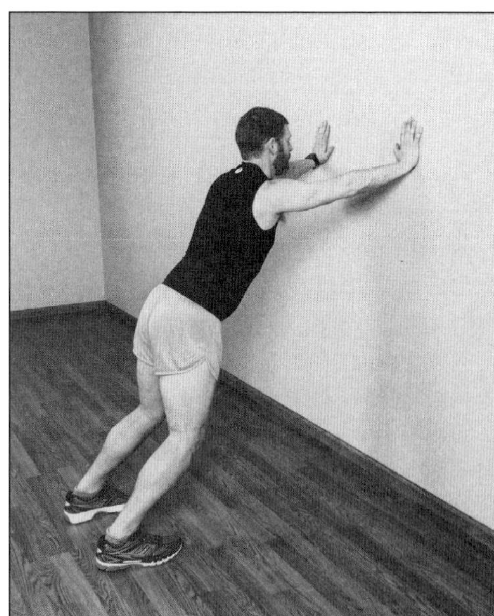

FIGURE 6.14 Soleus stretch with wall.

SOLEUS STRETCH WITHOUT WALL

1. Begin with the feet underneath the hips and the hands at the hips.
2. Inhale to slide the right foot back slowly, maintaining the foot forward, neutral position.
3. Exhale to press the right heel into the ground.
4. Inhale to bend the front left knee as necessary to feel the stretch through the calf.
5. Exhale to bend the right knee slightly, keeping that heel glued to the ground, to feel a stretch in the lower calf (figure 6.15).
6. Maintain position for 8 to 10 breath cycles.
7. Exhale and step the back foot forward to the starting position.
8. Repeat with the left leg.

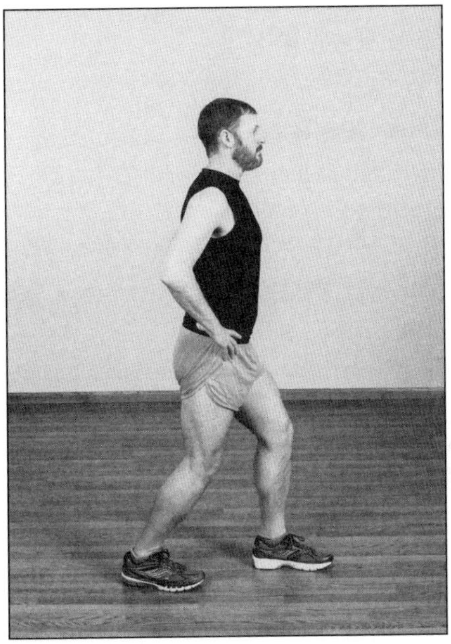

FIGURE 6.15 Soleus stretch without wall.

Consider This

The soleus stretch is intense. If only the gastrocnemius is stretched (straight-leg stretch), it will have little effect in increasing range of motion around the ankle joint, which is what is required to lengthen stride behind the body for a more effective toe push-off. The bent-knee calf stretch must be done to access the soleus.

Cues That Work

- Maintain a straight line from the heels (or the heel of the extended leg) to the crown of the head.
- Lift and spread the toes!
- Gently pull the navel toward the spine, *especially in stretches where no wall is used.*
- Breathe.
- Exhale to move into a slightly deeper stretch.

BACK OF UPPER LEG

Joints Targeted

Hips, knees

Muscles Targeted

Hamstring group including biceps femoris, semitendinosus, semimembranosus

HAMSTRING STRETCH WITH WALL

1. Stand facing a wall. Place the hands at shoulder height and width, arms straight, and keep the feet under the hips. (If a wall is not available, you can use a railing or tree.)
2. Inhale to hinge at the hips, reaching the chest toward the ground and keeping the head higher than the heart. It may be necessary to bend the arms or step the feet back to keep them under the hips as the torso lowers.
3. Stop the hinge movement when the stretch in the back of the upper legs becomes apparent (figure 6.16).
4. Maintain this position for 8 to 10 breath cycles.
5. Exhale to return to the starting position.

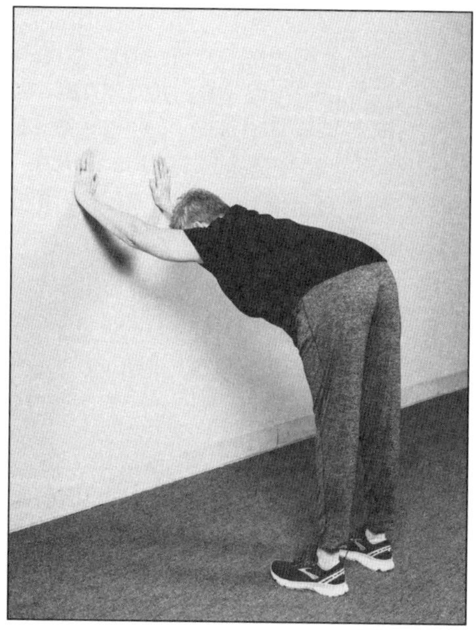

FIGURE 6.16 Hamstring stretch with wall.

HAMSTRING STRETCH WITHOUT WALL

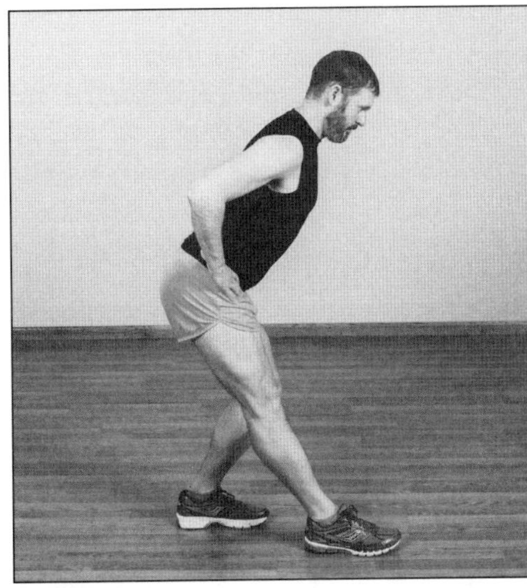

FIGURE 6.17 Hamstring stretch without wall.

1. Stand with the feet under the hips and the hands at the hips.
2. Inhale to step the right foot forward, placing the whole foot on the ground without moving the spine forward from its neutral position.
3. Exhale to hinge at the hips, try to maintain lumbar extension, and reach the chest toward the ground while visualizing the right hip pulling away from the right ankle. Keep the right leg straight. Hips need to be stacked over the back heel. The back leg needs to bend (as if sitting on an imaginary bench).
4. Stop the hinge movement when a stretch in the back of the upper right leg becomes apparent (figure 6.17).
5. Maintain this position for 8 to 10 breath cycles.
6. Inhale to stand up.
7. Exhale to return to starting position.
8. Repeat with left foot forward.

Consider This

A proper stretch of the hamstring group helps many people with low-back and piriformis problems. Here's how to maintain proper form to protect these areas while stretching.

- In both types of hamstring stretches, ensure that the natural lordotic curve of the low back stays in place. This is assisted by hinging at the hips rather than folding at the waist; a fold at the waist results in stretching of the low back rather than the hamstring group. Visualize lumbar spinal extension.
- In single-leg versions of this stretch, people tend to pull their toes toward their shins. While this still stretches the hamstring group, it may increase the calf stretch to such an extent that people lose a sense of stretching the hamstrings. Instead, let the foot relax naturally.
- In the single-leg versions, stand up straight before lifting the front foot to return to the starting position. This prevents strain on the low back.
- For an alternate single-leg, no-wall stretch, place the heel on an elevated curb or bench, foot relaxed. Many will feel the hamstring stretch immediately. If not, tell them to hinge the torso forward from the hips, keeping head and chest lifted.

Cues That Work

Wall Version

- Hinge at the hips.
- Aim the tailbone toward the sky.
- Keep the hands in place on the wall to maintain the natural curve in the low back.

No-Wall Version

- Hinge at the hips.
- Imagine sitting on an imaginary bench.
- Reach the chest forward.
- Pull the hip away from the heel.
- Return to standing before moving the front leg.

BUTTOCKS

Joints Targeted

Hips

Muscles Targeted

Gluteus maximus, gluteus medius, gluteus minimus, piriformis

GLUTE STRETCH WITH WALL

1. Stand facing a wall (or railing or tree), both feet a little closer than arm's-length away from the wall. Place both hands on the wall for balance. Shift the body weight over the left leg. Inhale and bend the right leg, resting the right ankle on the left thigh, above the left knee.
2. Exhale to flex the left hip and knee and lower into a one-leg squat, feeling the stretch through the right glutes (figure 6.18).
3. Hold for 8 to 10 breath cycles.
4. Inhale to straighten the left leg, lower the right foot to the ground, and return to the starting position.
5. Repeat steps 1 through 4 on the other leg.

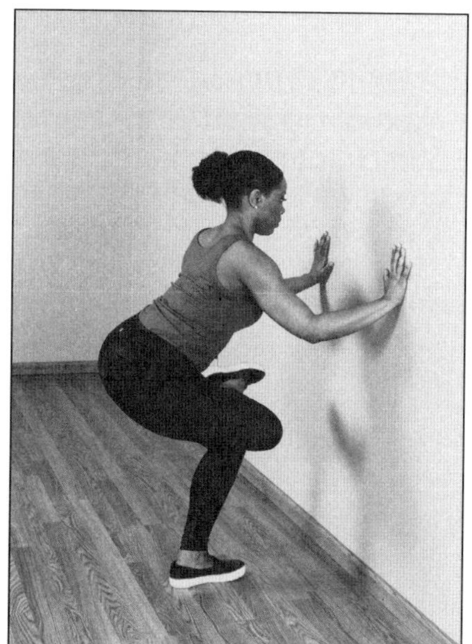

FIGURE 6.18 Glute stretch with wall.

SEATED GLUTE STRETCH

1. Sit on a bench with both legs extended in front of the body, heels resting on the ground. Inhale to lift the right leg and place the right ankle on the left thigh, above the left knee. Then, exhale to bend the left knee to 90 degrees, bringing the right ankle up higher. Place right hand to right inner thigh to emphasize external rotation of the hip joint (figure 6.19).
2. Inhale to lift through the spine and notice if there is a stretch through the glute area.
3. For a deeper stretch, inhale to hinge at the hips and reach the chest forward.
4. Maintain the stretch for 8 to 10 breath cycles.
5. Inhale to extend at the hips and return the spine to neutral as the right leg straightens, releasing the left foot to the ground to the starting position.
6. Repeat steps 1 to 5 with the opposite leg.

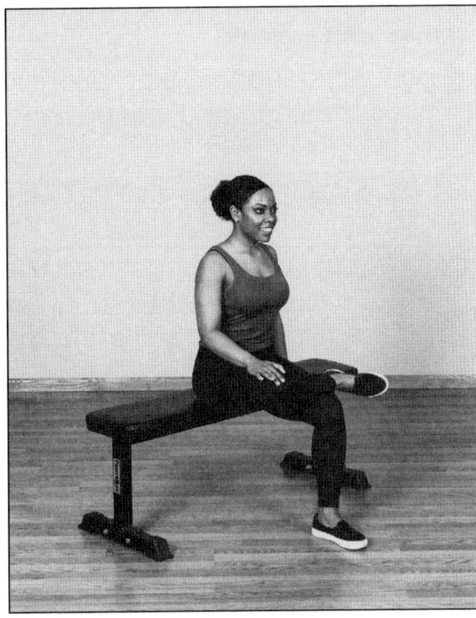

FIGURE 6.19 Glute stretch with bench.

Consider This

The piriformis often functions as a stabilizer, and repeated isometric muscle contractions can lead to delayed onset muscle soreness (DOMS), tightness, and inflammation. If not addressed, piriformis syndrome can develop, which manifests as pain in the sacroiliac joint and stiffness though the hip and low back. Because it is a common injury, you may have clients who complain of it. Performing glute stretches after a workout or even in the middle, if needed, can offer relief.

Cues That Work

- Keep the spine tall.
- Keep the rib cage lifted.
- Hinge at the hips rather than the waist.

FRONT OF UPPER LEG AND HIP

Joints Targeted

Hip, knee, lumbar spine

Muscles Targeted

Iliopsoas, quadriceps group including rectus femoris, vastus intermedius, vastus medialis, and vastus lateralis

QUADRICEPS STRETCH WITH WALL

1. Stand with the right side of the body next to a wall, with the feet under the hips. Place the right hand on the wall for balance, with the left arm hanging at the side. (If a wall is not available, use a railing or tree.)
2. Inhale to bend the left knee and bring the left foot up into the left hand.
3. Exhale to line up both knees to feel a stretch in the front of the hip and thigh (figure 6.20).
4. For a deeper stretch, inhale to keep the spine tall and gently press the left hip forward.
5. Maintain this position for 8 to 10 breath cycles.
6. Exhale to return to the starting position.
7. Repeat steps 1 to 6 with the opposite leg.

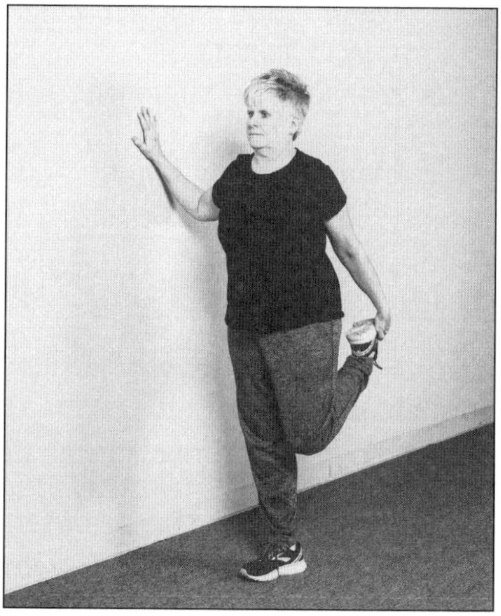

FIGURE 6.20 Quadriceps stretch with wall.

QUADRICEPS STRETCH WITHOUT WALL

1. Stand with the feet under the hips. Shift body weight to the left leg. While inhaling, place the right leg behind the body with the top of the foot and toenails touching and facing the ground.
2. On the next inhalation, bring the hands to the low back and lift the chest toward the sky as the head relaxes back. Feel a stretch in the front of the hip and thigh (figure 6.21).
3. Maintain this position for 8 to 10 breath cycles.
4. Exhale to return to the starting position.
5. Repeat with the left leg behind.

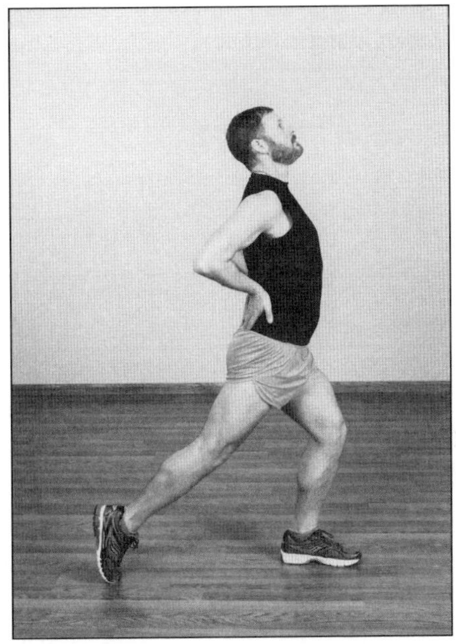

FIGURE 6.21 Quadriceps stretch without wall.

Consider This

While walking is good at moving the hip flexor group out of flexion, most people benefit from additional stretching of the anterior hip muscles, tendons, and ligaments that are shortened from hours of sitting. This also improves walking performance by allowing the stride length to increase behind the body.

- Encourage a tall spine to promote opening through the front of the hip. Many people tend to fold forward at the hip and waist, which negates the stretch. The spine should also be in a neutral position to avoid overarching the low back during the wall version.
- Since curbs are often available in walking classes, you can utilize them for an alternative no-wall version of the stretch. With back to the curb, place the back foot over the curb (top of the foot and toes on the curb) to add to the opening of the anterior hip.

Cues That Work

- Line up the knees in wall version.
- Stand tall: Visualize the crown of the head reaching to the sky in the wall version.
- Use the hands to support the low back in no-wall version as the top of the back foot presses toward the ground.
- Gently press the hip of the bent leg forward to maximize the anterior hip stretch in wall version.

SHIN

Joint Targeted

Ankle

Muscles Targeted

Tibialis anterior, peroneus longus, peroneus brevis, and peroneus tertius

SHIN STRETCH

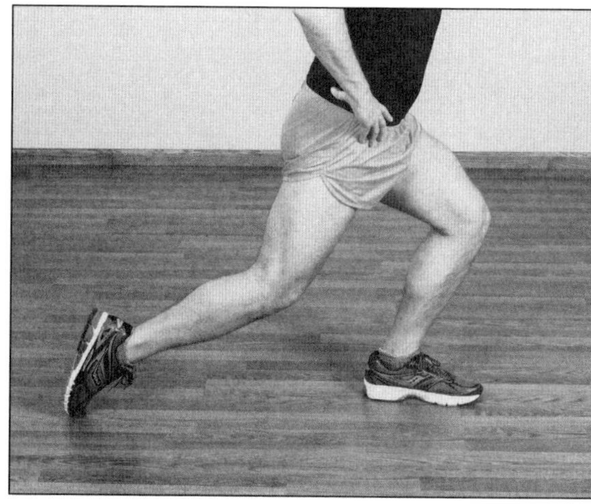

FIGURE 6.22 Shin stretch.

1. Stand tall, with the hands at the hips. Shift the body weight over the left foot and leg. Inhale and step the right foot behind, pointing the toes and placing them on the ground so the toenails and top of the foot faces down on the ground.
2. Exhale to press the top of the toes and foot toward the ground so that a stretch is felt in the shin area (figure 6.22).
3. Maintain this position for 8 to 10 breath cycles.
4. Keeping the foot pointed behind the body, let the right ankle fall away from midline to stretch the peroneal group.
5. Maintain this position for 8 to 10 breath cycles.
6. Exhale to return to the starting position.
7. Repeat with the left leg.

Consider This

Stretching the tibialis anterior improves walking performance by releasing the ankle for greater posterior range of motion during the toe push-off. It is a difficult muscle to stretch and some people may find it easier to achieve a stretch through this area while barefoot. If it is unusually tight, clients may want to regularly kneel on their shins at home as a way of stretching or try massage for this area.

Cues That Work

- Make sure the toenails are directed toward the ground.
- Press the whole top of the foot toward the ground.
- Press the hip of that leg forward.

Upper Body

CHEST, SHOULDERS, AND ARMS

Joints Targeted

Thoracic spine, shoulders

Muscles Targeted

Pectoralis major, pectoralis minor, serratus anterior, coracobrachialis, biceps brachii, subscapularis

PEC STRETCH

1. Stand with the front of the body against a wall, with the right arm raised parallel to the ground and the palm touching the wall.
2. Inhale to keep the right arm in position and exhale to slowly peel the body away from the wall, moving the feet so that they turn away from the wall.
3. Feel the stretch in the right biceps, right shoulder, and chest (figure 6.23).
4. Maintain this position for 8 to 10 breath cycles.
5. Exhale to return to face the wall to return to starting position.
6. Repeat on the left side.

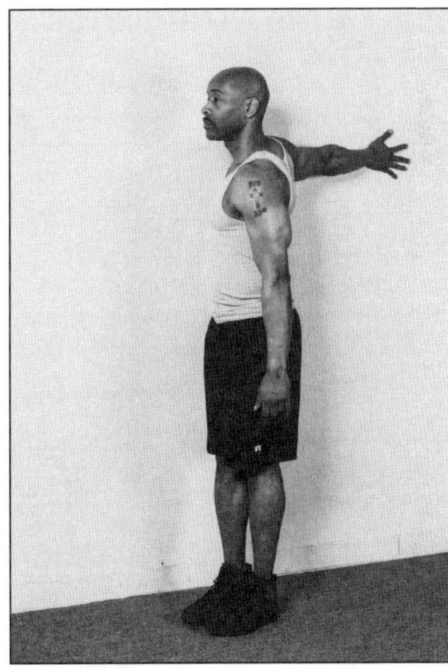

FIGURE 6.23 Pec stretch with a wall.

Consider This

Many people are tight across the chest and front of the shoulders because of occupational and leisure activities that cause them to round forward—looking at phones, working at computers, and driving cars—so it is important to stretch this area regularly. For additional stretches that you can give to your clients to do at home, see the Releasing the Chest Muscles for Better Posture section later in this chapter. In class, stretching the chest and shoulders in the standing position is often easiest with a wall, tree, pole, or even a partner. Here are ways to vary the stretch.

- The arm can be placed higher or lower on the wall to target different muscle fibers in the chest, shoulders, and arms.

- Bend the arms at the elbows to focus more on the muscles of the chest.
- If there is no wall or tree available, partner your clients into pairs and have them press their arms against each other instead of a wall.

Cues That Work

- Stand tall.
- Move slowly.
- Keep breathing.

Releasing the Chest Muscles for Better Posture

A tall posture radiates strength and youthfulness. It also improves the ability of a walker to recruit the muscles of the posterior chain to power their walk. Because so much of daily life is spent in spinal flexion (forward lean or bend), the muscles of the chest and fronts of the shoulders become shortened and tight. This restricts the ability to stand tall. To counteract the effects of so much time in spinal flexion, a daily routine of stretching across the chest and shoulders makes sense. Here are two exercises that your clients can do at home to complement the stretching they do with you in class.

DOORFRAME CHEST STRETCH

1. Stand in the middle of a standard doorway, the feet under the hips and arms bent at 90 degrees in "goal post" position, resting on the door frame.
2. Inhale to lean the chest and body forward until a stretch is felt across the chest and front of shoulders (figure 6.24).
3. Maintain this position for 8 to 10 breath cycles.
4. Exhale to return to start position.

This stretch can also be done with the arms overheard and hands touching the top of the door frame. If the doorway is wide, the arms can be extended out to the side, with the forearms or hands holding the sides of the door frame.

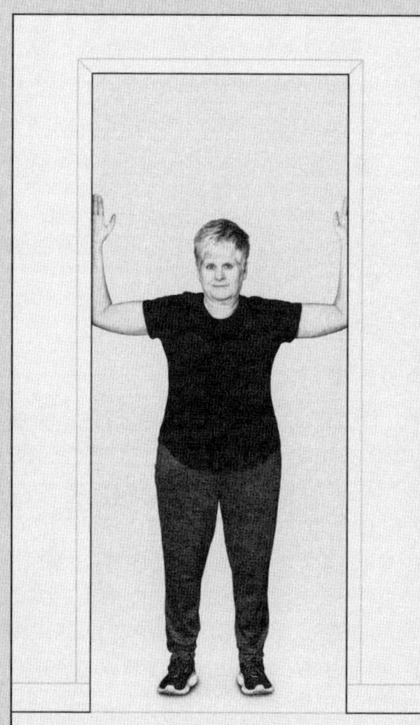

FIGURE 6.24 Door frame chest stretch.

SUPINE CHEST STRETCH

1. Roll up a blanket so that it is no wider than the space between the inside edges of the shoulder blades (about 2-3 in. [5-8 cm]), long enough to run from the center of the back of the head to the spine just below the shoulder blades (about 16-18 in. [41-36 cm]), and about three inches (9 cm) high from the floor. (A bolster with similar dimensions can be used.)
2. Sit with the low back at one end of the blanket or bolster, knees bent and soles of the feet on the floor.
3. Exhale to slowly lie back on the blanket so that it connects at the spine below the shoulder blades, up to the back of the head.
4. Inhale to straighten the legs and open the arms wide to rest on the floor beside the body, with the palms facing the ceiling (figure 6.25). If the arms cannot rest on the floor, the blanket or bolster is too high.
5. Maintain this position for 8 to 10 breaths.
6. To exit, gently bend the knees and roll off to one side before sitting up.

As the body becomes more comfortable with this stretch, the range of motion can be increased by using a rolled-up blanket or bolster that is higher from the ground so that the arch in the back is more pronounced.

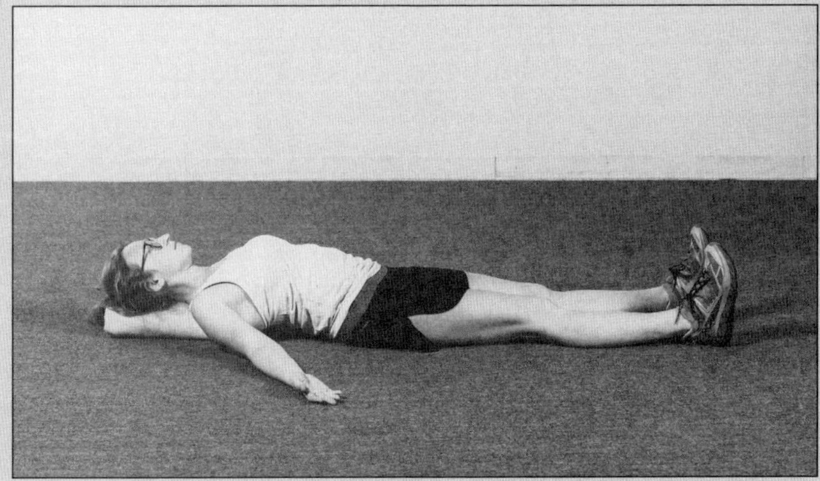

FIGURE 6.25 Supine chest stretch.

Starting off with the dynamic stretch routine included in this chapter will ensure your class participants or clients will be ready to get the most out of the walking workout. Finish with the postworkout performance stretches to increase range of motion around the joints that result in long-term increases in walking speed and improve posture—a huge take-home benefit to health and a sense of well-being. In the next chapter, you will learn strength training techniques to create a comprehensive walking fitness routine and help your clients build strength and endurance.

References

1. Small, K., McNaughton, L., and Matthews, M. 2008. "A Systematic Review Into the Efficacy of Static Stretching as Part of a Warm-Up for the Prevention of Exercise-Related Injury." *Research in Sports Medicine* 16 (3): 213–31. doi: 10.1080/15438620802310784.
2. Fradkin, A.J., Zazryn, T.R., and Smoliga, J.M. 2010. "Effects of Warming-Up on Physical Performance: A Systemic Review With Meta-Analysis." *Journal of Strength and Conditioning Research* 24 (1): 140-48. doi: 10.1519/JSC.0b013e3181c643a0.
3. Page, P. 2012. "Current Concepts in Muscle Stretching for Exercise and Rehabilitation." *International Journal of Sports and Physical Therapy* 7 (1): 109-19.

7

Gain Strength for Power

Introducing your walking clients to strength training is an opportunity to witness great success. Strengthening exercises can be incorporated easily into outdoor walking classes or encouraged as home practice. With a small investment of time, strength training results in a plethora of physical improvements, including the ability to perform daily tasks with greater ease, relatively fast and noticeable body changes, quicker walking speeds, and a sense of greater stability around the joints.

Many people know that they should be getting about 30 minutes of cardio exercise (walking, running, swimming, cycling) at least five days a week. That's probably why they are coming to your walking classes or groups. But for many, another important physical activity guideline probably isn't on their radar. All adults should be doing muscle-strengthening exercises for all the major muscle groups twice a week. While 52 percent of American adults did enough cardio exercise to meet that recommendation in 2016, only 22 percent met both recommendations, according to the latest data released from the National Center for Health Statistics [1]. And considering the demographic that favors walking, typically those over age 30, it would be a disservice to not encourage them to do some type of strength training.

Muscle mass begins to decline at a rate of one to two percent a year around age 30. This consistent loss adds up year after year and accelerates as we age, until it becomes noticeably harder to do everyday activities, including walking. In a 2004 Swedish study, researchers found that decreases in lower-body muscle strength resulted in poor walking performance even in healthy people, according to research published in the *Archives of Physical Medicine and Rehabilitation* [2]. The lower percentage of muscle in the body also affects metabolism, making it easier to gain weight. These added pounds exacerbate the difficulties of being active already happening because of strength loss. Strength training can attenuate this muscle loss and even help to rebuild muscle mass at any age.

Strength training improves resting metabolic rate (RMR), bone density near the muscles being strengthened, insulin sensitivity, and range of motion around joints. It also reduces risk of diabetes, eases joint pain, and helps manage osteoarthritis, and it is now being credited with reducing symptoms of depression. With such an expansive and diverse set of benefits, it makes sense that walking performance, too, can be enhanced by a strength training program. Strong muscles support joint stability for aerobic activity and power the workout so that it is more effective. In a 2015 meta-analysis published in *BMC Geriatrics*, researchers in the Netherlands identified progressive resistance training as the most effective exercise modality at improving gait speed [3].

Specifically targeting the muscles of the posterior chain will also help to counteract everyday habits that create postural challenges to walking more powerfully and faster. Whether you have clients who are active or sedentary, the occupational and leisure activities of our society such as sitting at desks for work and watching screens for entertainment result in spines positioned in constant flexion. As they sit in front of computers, look at cell phones, and drive cars, the muscles of the posterior chain, which are the key focus of the walking technique progressions, become overstretched, and anterior muscles shorten. Not only does this create poor posture in people, it also means that those stretched muscles of the posterior chain are weak and offer minimal power to drive the walk. With a strength training program that focuses on the posterior chain muscles, your clients can reverse this. For example, as back muscles such as the latissimus dorsi and rhomboids are strengthened, chest muscles are stretched, including the pectoralis and even the anterior deltoids. These changes pull people into an improved and more upright posture that enhances overall appearance and better powers walking.

Additionally, strengthening all the stabilizer muscles attached to the hips, knees, and ankles will lower risk for injury at these joints. In a society where we are not only sitting for long periods but also inactive, we need our joints to be supported when we do get up and move.

And the benefits of strength training go beyond just the physical. Seeing improvements in the body, often more quickly than with cardio exercise, increases confidence and self-esteem. In a Montana State University study [4], 341 women between the ages of 23 and 87 did a strength training class twice a week for about 10 weeks. Afterward, they enjoyed all types of physical activity more and became more active throughout the day. They also reported significantly improved body images. Similar effects have been shown with men as well [5].

Incorporating Strength in Walking Class

We have found that our clients arrive to walking class with a variety of fitness experience. For many, a fitness program means a cardio workout. We agree this should be the priority, because research shows that consistently challenging the heart to a workout lowers risk for most disease. While cardio is what your clients may be coming to you for, given the general health benefits and specific improvements to walking speed that strength training has to offer, you should be an advocate for strength training, too.

Once your clients have discovered the feel-good effects of walking in class, you have set up a bond of trust that allows you to introduce strength training into your programming. Then, you can share all the benefits of

Worksite Walking

Case Study

As corporate fitness manager at a large multicampus business, Laura Locker is always searching for innovative ways to attract employees to work out and motivate them to keep coming back. That's one of the reasons Laura regularly attends the ACSM's annual Health & Fitness Summit. The corporate gym at the head office has good attendance for classes, but it's usually the same faces.

That changed after the 2014 summit when Laura attended Michele and Lee's walking workout session. She was inspired to bring outdoor walking to her company fitness program to entice employees who weren't currently motivated by typical class programming.

Laura introduced lunchtime walking programs that featured interval training in summer and fall in three different ways: a free eight-week pilot project geared specifically to nonmembers and focused more on enjoying exercise, an outdoor walking workout class within the drop-in group fitness programming, and an eight-week fee-based class limited to 10 participants to allow more personal coaching to improve their performance.

Using technology to her advantage, Locker invited nonmembers of the corporate gym to join the initial pilot project for no charge if they agreed to use MapMyFitness as a tracking tool. If a person missed class, they would have to do a "home walk" while logged in to MapMyFitness so that Locker could confirm attendance. Thanks to the walking programs, employees who previously shied away from the corporate fitness center were now showing up for classes and being more active. The walking classes also offered more variety for those who were already working out.

While there are no specific walking workout classes at the company's regional offices, Locker has offered multiple single-session workshops on good walking form, averaging about 20 participants each time. The company offers step incentive programs, such as this year's challenge encouraging people to walk 3,000,000 steps or more during the year to be eligible for monetary awards. Laura has seen people walking the halls using the power-walking technique they learned in these workshops to accrue steps.

"Walking is a physical activity that checks all the boxes," says Locker. It can be done with any amount of time, at any time, and it requires limited equipment. "We always have our feet with us," she says. It also has the added benefit of being done outside, which is a draw for some. And for others who may be intimidated by gym settings, they can avoid the gym while still getting a good workout.

strength training, adding another layer of physical challenge to expand fitness as well as a sense of accomplishment and well-being.

People who enjoy an outdoor walking workout often appreciate incorporating strength training in that outdoor environment. The seven exercises included here can be done easily while outside. The program utilizes body weight because it is always with you and resistance bands because they are inexpensive and portable. The coach can carry the resistance bands in a small pack, or walkers can carry them. Typically, people will need two resistance levels of bands: less resistance for smaller muscles and greater resistance for larger muscles.

Resistance training can be introduced in walking classes in many ways. If you have the luxury of 60- to 90-minute classes, take 15 minutes before the cool-down stroll and stretches to lead some of the exercises shown in this chapter. Alternatively, you may find there is interest in holding one or two classes a week dedicated to strength training. If you live in a place that experiences cold, snowy, or icy winters, put away the bands during that time to focus on body-weight training. In these cold conditions, the bands can snap, leaving people vulnerable to painful injury. (Even if you live where it is warm year-round, always check bands before class for signs of deterioration, and throw them away immediately at the first sign of tears or thinning of the band.)

Remind clients that amazing gains in muscle strength will happen with just a couple of sessions per week, when muscles are challenged to a point of fatigue and then given a chance to recover from the work-to-fatigue session. The opportunity to repair and build is crucial. Encourage slow movement without momentum to recruit all muscle fibers. Always emphasize good form, especially for people new to strength training. In the words of legendary coach Vince Lombardi, only "perfect practice makes perfect."

Walkers will directly benefit from strength training targeted to several specific muscle groups, including propulsive muscles (the muscles that move the body forward) of the buttocks (glutes), back of the upper leg (hamstring group, including semitendinosus and biceps of the femur), back of shoulders (posterior deltoid, infraspinatus, teres major and minor, latissimus dorsi, rhomboids), and the calf (gastrocnemius, soleus).

Braking muscles and stabilizing muscles (the muscles that stop or slow the body down and help resist falling) should also be worked, including those in the back of the upper leg (hamstring group), on the outside of the upper leg (tensor fasciae latae, gluteus medius, vastus medialis, vastus lateralis), in the front of the upper leg (quadriceps group, including rectus femoris and adductor), and the front and side of the shin (tibialis anterior, peroneal group). All muscles do not need equal attention because they work in different ways while walking, depending on the phase of the gait.

We encourage a progressive approach to teaching strength exercises, just as we do for walking, so that there are options for success at several levels. Keep these points in mind when instructing walkers.

- Using bands, always start with a band that is easy. It is much better for people to learn the movement with little resistance or possibly no band at all. Gradually increase resistance until they find a band that allows them to successfully complete 8 to 12 repetitions to fatigue. Typically, people will need a band offering more resistance for the leg exercises, and bands offering less resistance for the upper-body work.

- In addition to using another band with more or less resistance, the amount of resistance can be adjusted by changing hand position. Moving hands closer together or closer to the point of attachment will increase resistance. Moving them farther apart or away from the attachment point will create more slack in the band and decrease resistance.
- Aim to do 1 to 3 sets of each exercise with a 30- to 90-second rest in between if performing all of the sets of an exercise back to back.
- Explain to clients that they can identify fatigue when there is a temptation to hold the breath or it is tough to maintain good form. Encourage them to pay attention to the moment when breath and good form are being sacrificed.
- If they don't notice fatigue by the last rep of the last set of an exercise, then they need to use a band with more resistance or shorten the length of the band that they are using to create more resistance.
- People often hold their breath when any exercise gets difficult. Watch for this. Advise when to inhale and when to exhale. We suggest cuing "exhale on exertion." Also note that when we speak, we automatically exhale, so you can suggest people count repetitions aloud on the exertion phase of the exercise.

LUNGES

Muscles Targeted

Prime movers: hamstring and gluteus maximus, quadriceps

Additional muscles targeted (walking lunge with twist): oblique abdominals

Synergists and stabilizers: gluteus medius and minimus, oblique abdominals

STATIONARY LUNGE

1. Stand tall, feet hip-width apart and hands on hips. Step the right foot back as far as possible. The right heel should be off the floor so weight is on the ball of the right foot and toes (figure 7.1*a*).
2. Inhale while bending the knees and lowering the body straight down until the left thigh is parallel to the ground (figure 7.1*b*).
3. Exhale while pressing into both feet, straighten the legs, and raise the body to the starting position.
4. Do 8 to 12 repetitions, inhaling to lower and exhaling to rise. On the last rep, push off with the back foot and return to standing with feet together.
5. Repeat with the left foot back.

(continued)

STATIONARY LUNGE *(continued)*

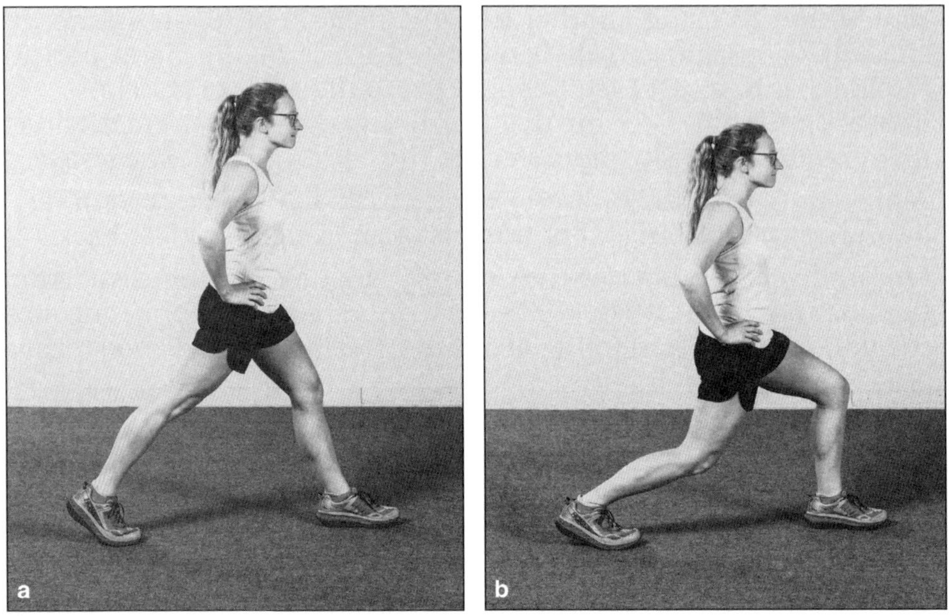

FIGURE 7.1 Stationary lunge: *(a)* start position and *(b)* down position.

BACK LUNGE

1. Stand tall, feet hip-width distance apart and hands on hips.
2. Inhale while stepping the right foot back as far as possible, landing on the ball and toes of the right foot, the right heel off the ground. Immediately bend the knees and lower the body straight down until the left thigh is parallel to the ground.
3. Exhale while pushing off with the back foot, and return to standing with the feet together.
4. Repeat stepping left foot back and alternating legs for all reps, or do all repetitions with the right foot and then repeat with the left foot.
5. Do 8 to 12 repetitions on each side.

STEP-TOGETHER TRAVELING LUNGE

1. Stand tall, feet hip-width apart and hands on hips.
2. Inhale while stepping the right foot forward as far as possible and lifting the left heel off the ground, coming up onto the ball and toes of the back left foot. Immediately bend the knees and lower the body straight down until the right thigh is parallel to the ground.
3. Maintain good contact between the heel of the right foot and the ground, exhale to push off with the left foot. Step the left foot forward bringing it next to the right foot.

4. Alternate the right and left foot stepping forward, or do all repetitions with the right foot and then repeat with the left foot.
5. Do 8 to 12 repetitions on each side.

WALKING LUNGE

1. Stand tall, feet hip-width apart and hands on hips.
2. Inhale while stepping the right foot forward as far as possible. Lifting the left heel off the ground, come up onto the ball and toes of the left back foot. Immediately bend the knees and lower the body straight down until the right thigh is parallel to the ground.
3. Maintain good contact with heel of the right foot and the ground, and exhale to push off with the left foot. Swing the left foot all the way through, taking a step forward, and then immediately bending the knees and lowering into a lunge.
4. Repeat, pushing off with and stepping the right foot forward. Continue alternating legs.
5. Do 8 to 12 repetitions on each side.

WALKING LUNGE WITH TWIST

1. Stand tall, feet hip-width apart and hands on hips.
2. Inhale while stepping the right foot forward as far as possible, coming up onto the ball and toes of the back left foot with the left heel off the ground. Immediately bend the knees and lower the body straight down until the right thigh is parallel to the ground.
3. In the lunge position, exhale to bring the left hand across the body to the outside of the right thigh, twisting the torso to the right (figure 7.2).
4. Inhale while rotating the torso back to center.
5. Maintain good contact between the heel of the right foot and the ground, exhale to push off with the left foot. Swing the left foot all the way through, taking a step forward, and then immediately bending the knees, lowering into a lunge, and twisting to the left (right hand across to the outside of the left thigh).
6. Repeat stepping the right foot forward and continue, alternating legs.
7. Do 8 to 12 repetitions on each side.

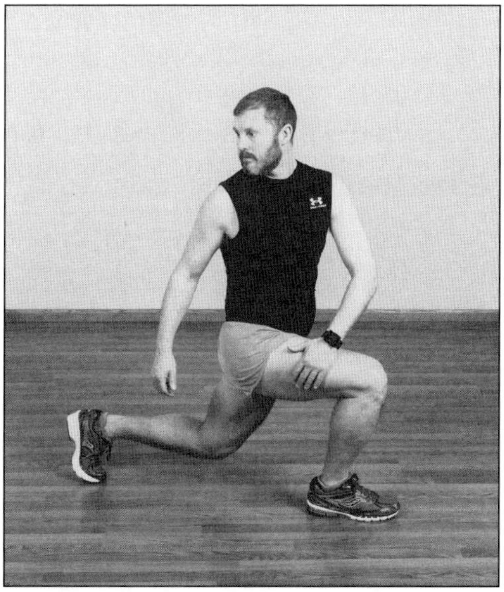

FIGURE 7.2 Walking lunge with twist.

Consider This

Keep an eye out for these common misalignments that make the exercise unnecessarily difficult and pose risk for injury.

- *Burning quads or knee pain*—If clients feel the work through the quadriceps group only or experience pain in the knee, the forward stride for the lunge is too short and weight is shifting too far forward over the ball of the foot (the angle of the knee is smaller than 90 degrees). Check that the knee of the front leg is in alignment with the ankle of that same leg and encourage people to test this by lifting their toes in their shoes to ensure stability in that position. The tendency to carry too much weight into the front of the foot results in poor muscle recruitment of the glutes and hamstrings and poses risk for injury to the knee and/or falling from the resulting instability. The easiest way to correct this common error is to lengthen the stride by wiggling the rear foot farther back.
- *Off balance*—Ensure that the feet are maintaining a hip-width distance even in the lunge position. A helpful cue for this is to imagine standing on a wood deck with feet hip-width apart and each foot on a separate wooden plank. Whether they step forward or back to assume the lunge position, the foot lands on its own wooden plank.

Increase the Challenge

When your clients have mastered these moves, here are suggestions to increase the challenge without progressing to another variation:

- *Double dip*—At the low point of the lunge, rise a little and then lower back down before coming all the way back up.
- *Add weight*—You could encourage clients to do these lunges on their own at home while holding weights at their sides. The weights could be as simple as cans of tomatoes!
- *Go vertical*—Try doing walking lunges up an incline to emphasize glute work. Walk normally on the decline because walking lunges downhill would put the knee at risk for injury.

Cues That Work

- Be bold! Step far back or step far forward to protect the knees.
- Lift the heel of the back foot so that a long stance is possible.
- Keep hip-width distance between the two feet by keeping each foot on its wooden plank.
- Can you see the toes of your front foot? They need to be visible beyond the knee of that same leg at all times.
- Keep the front heel glued into the ground.
- Maintain a tall spine. Eyes to the horizon!
- Squeeze the glutes of the front leg to "scissor" the legs together when performing any lunge variation that requires a toe push-off.

Lunge With Less Risk

Coaching Tip

You may notice that a common front lunge variation, in which the person steps forward with one foot into the lunge and then pushes off with the front foot to return backward to standing, is not part of the progression above. In practice, we have found that people often experience knee pain when doing this variation, even if their form is excellent. Instead, the variations we offer here work to strengthen the targeted muscles without the risk of pain or injury.

SQUATS

Muscles Targeted

Prime movers: erector spinae, gluteus maximus, quadriceps femoris, rectus femoris, vastus intermedius, vastus medialis, hamstring group (including semitendinosus, semimembranosus, biceps femoris)

Synergists and stabilizers: transversus abdominis, gluteus medius and minimus, adductors, soleus, gastrocnemius

Equipment

Resistance band and bench for variations

BENCH RISE

1. Sit at the edge of a bench at a height allowing the thighs to be parallel to the ground or higher. Feet should be flat on the ground and hip-width apart. Place the hands on the bench on either side of the hips or at the low back (figure 7.3*a*).
2. Exhale while rooting the heels and soles of the feet into the ground, pulling the navel toward the spine, hinging at the hips, and pressing up to standing (figure 7.3*b*). (Hands can be used to assist with this lift or placed at sacral area for low-back support.)
3. Inhale to hinge forward at the hips and bend the knees to sit back down.
4. Do 8 to 12 repetitions.

(continued)

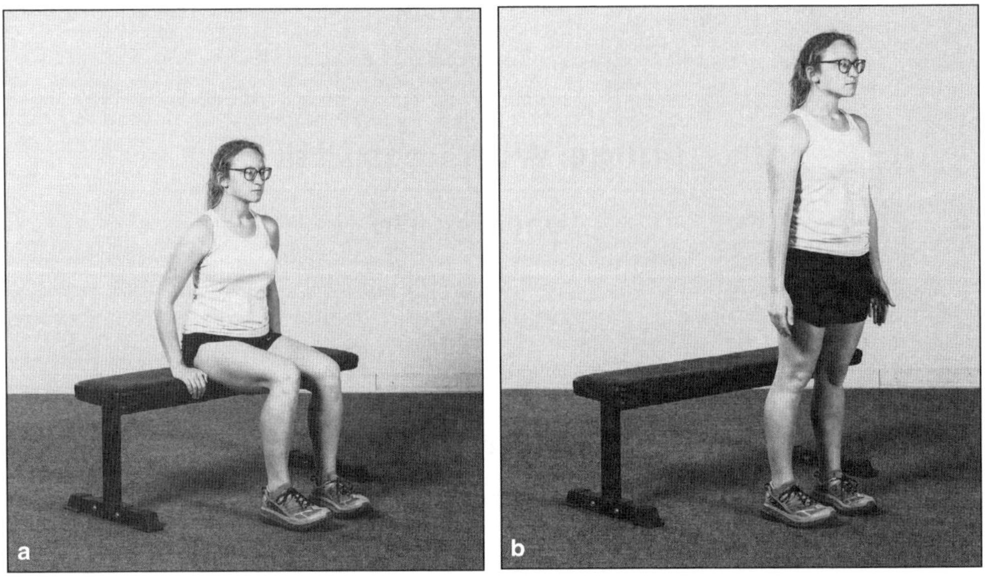

FIGURE 7.3 Bench rise: *(a)* starting position and *(b)* mid position.

BASIC SQUAT

1. Stand tall, feet hip-width apart and hands on hips or at the low back.
2. Inhale while flexing the hips and knees to lower, as if sitting back into a chair. Keep the heels and soles of the feet firmly rooted into the ground, body weight supported over the heels and the rib cage lifted. Arms can be extended in front to help with balance. Lower as far as possible while maintaining good form but not past thighs parallel to the ground (figure 7.4).
3. Exhale while pressing into the ground, straightening the legs and returning to standing.

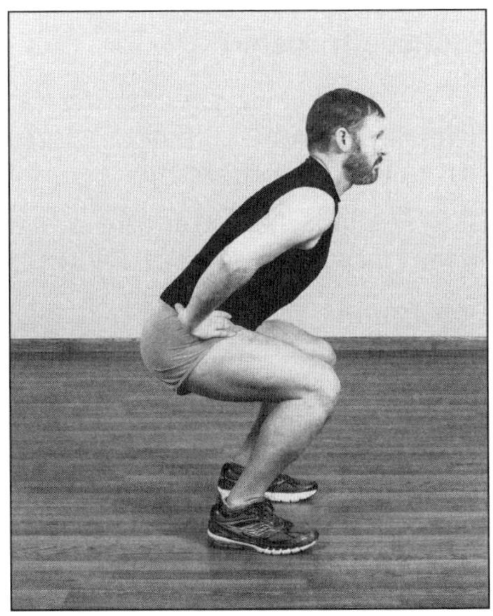

FIGURE 7.4 Basic squat.

SIDE-STEP MOVING SQUAT

1. Stand tall, feet together and hands on hips or at the low back.
2. Inhale while stepping the right foot out to the right side slightly wider than shoulder width, planting the right heel and sole of the foot into the ground.
3. Flex the hips and knees while lowering into a basic squat. Arms can be extended in front to help with balance.
4. Exhale while pressing into the ground, straightening the legs and stepping the left foot in beside the right foot to return to the standing position.
5. Do 8 to 12 repetitions leading with the right leg.
6. Repeat 8 to 12 repetitions leading with the left leg.

SIDE-STEP MOVING SQUAT WITH RESISTANCE BAND

1. Place a looped resistance band around the lower legs with feet separated enough to keep mild tension in the band.
2. Inhale while stepping the right foot out to the right side slightly wider than shoulder width, planting the right heel and sole of the foot into the ground.
3. Flex the hips and knees while lowering into a basic squat (figure 7.5).
4. Exhale while pressing into the ground, straightening the legs, and stepping the left foot in to start position, keeping tension in the band so that it does not fall to the ankles.
5. Do 8 to 12 repetitions leading with right leg.
6. Repeat 8 to 12 repetitions leading with left leg.

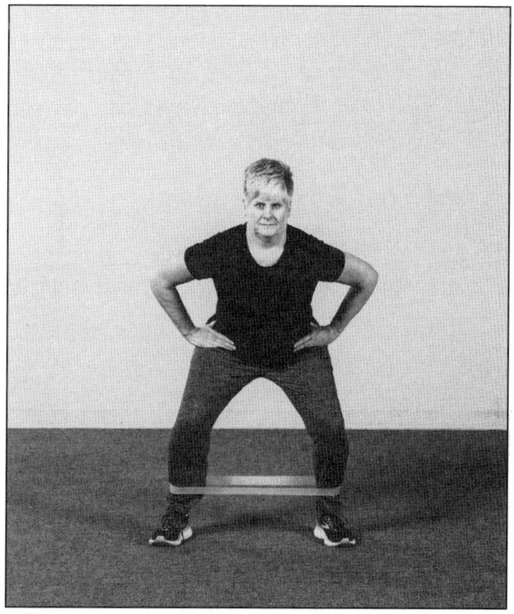

FIGURE 7.5 Side step moving squat with resistance band.

Consider This

The squat targets many leg muscles similar to those of lunging. We include it in our list of best practice exercises because, in addition to targeting propulsive muscles used for walking, it is highly functional for daily living. Keep an eye out for these common misalignments so that clients get the most from their workout.

- *Form matters*—Just like in the lunge, it is worth spending time to ensure that everyone discovers their best basic squat as any progression will be safer and easier. Sitting and coming up from seated is an activity repeated many times throughout a day, often without much thought or focus on form. Training for automatic good squat technique reduces the risk for low-back injury whenever squatting is a part of an everyday activity.
- *Check in*—Most of the cues reflect the key points that reinforce good form but often cuing is not enough for a movement that is repeated frequently during the day. Watch for good spinal extension, knees positioned over feet or behind the toes, and loading of body weight through the heels. Many people find the squat easiest with the hands and arms forward as they lower.

Progression

- Hold the low squat position for one or two breath cycles or vary timing of the up-and-down movements. For example, lower for four counts and rise for two counts.

Cues That Work

- Visualize hinging from hips; chest reaching forward.
- Sit in an imaginary chair as the hips lower.
- Root through the heels to rise.
- Maintain back extension.
- Lift your rib cage.
- Navel pulls toward spine.
- Knees track over and in the same direction as the feet.
- Toes should be visible while squatting. Extend arms in front if there is any feeling of instability.

STANDING LEG ADDUCTION/ABDUCTION

Adduction Muscles Targeted

Prime movers: pectineus, adductor brevis, adductor longus, adductor magnus, gracilis

Synergists and stabilizers: obturator externus, piriformis, obturator internus, quadratus femoris, pelvic floor muscles, transversus abdominis, rectus femoris, multifidi

Abduction Muscles Targeted

Prime movers: gluteus medius, tensor fasciae latae

Synergists and stabilizers: gluteus maximus, gluteus minimus, sartorius, piriformis, pelvic floor muscles, transversus abdominis, rectus femoris, multifidi

Equipment

Resistance band; heavy object, wall, or railing

STANDING LEG ADDUCTION AND ABDUCTION WITH RESISTANCE BAND

1. Anchor one end of a resistance band to a heavy object at ankle height and tie the other end around the lower right leg just above the ankle. Stand with the right side of the body toward where the band is attached. *Optional:* Place the right hand on a wall or railing for stability.
2. Exhale while pulling the right leg, with the foot in neutral, across the front of the body to midline or beyond (adduction) (figure 7.6*a*).
3. Inhale while returning to the start position. Do 8 to 12 repetitions.
4. Leaving the right foot in the resistance band, turn the whole body 180 degrees so that the right foot with the band is on the outside of the body relative to where the band is attached.
5. Exhale while pressing the right leg, with the foot in neutral, out to the side as far as possible, away from the anchor point (abduction) (figure 7.6*b*).
6. Inhale while returning the leg to the starting position. Do 8 to 12 repetitions.
7. Repeat the entire sequence of adduction and abduction using the left leg.

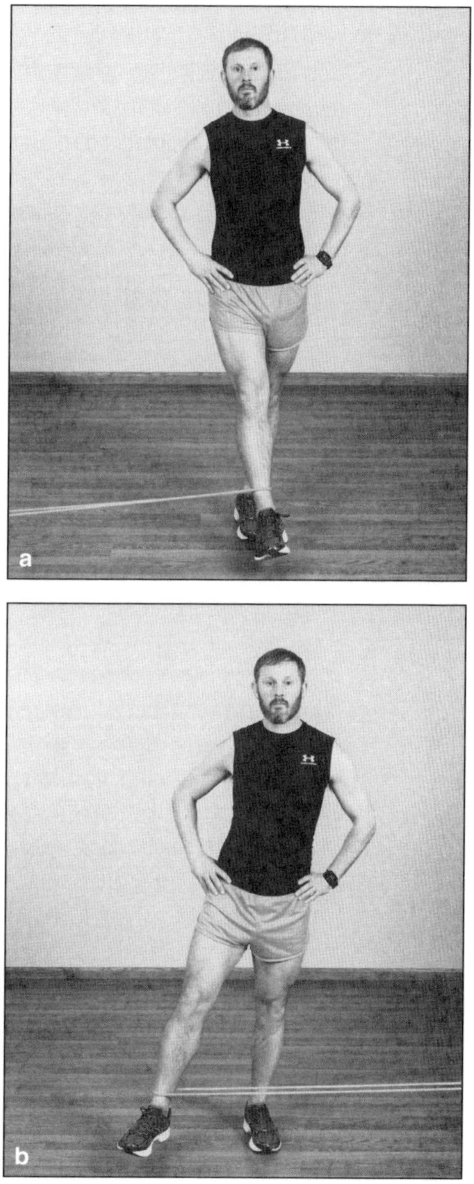

FIGURE 7.6 *(a)* Standing leg adduction; *(b)* standing leg abduction.

(continued)

STANDING LEG ADDUCTION AND ABDUCTION *(continued)*

Standing Leg Adduction and Abduction Variations

- Increase the resistance of the band.
- Turn the toes out, away from the midline, as the leg pulls across during adduction (figure 7.7*a*), and in toward the midline as the leg goes out to the side during abduction (figure 7.7*b*).
- Change the count pace. Consider slowing either the inhalation or exhalation phases: Inhale for half the time of the exhale phase, or inhale for double the time of the exhale phase.
- To challenge stability, place the hands at the waist without holding on to anything. A lighter resistance band is recommended when using this variation.

Consider This

- Many consider adduction and abduction exercises as targeting the muscles of the inner and outer thigh. This is true, but they can also work the core and pelvic floor muscles in a way that is highly functional for most people. If a walker feels comfortable and confident incorporating progression 4, hip rotation (see chapter 4), into their walking technique, just before the heel strike, the leg tracks slightly toward the midline. Strong adductor muscles will protect the knee during the braking of this heel strike. The reality is that most people have weak adductors and gluteus medius muscles. This exercise helps both!
- For clients who have come to you from running because of knee injury, strengthening these adductor and abductor muscles offers a powerful stabilizing effect on the knee.

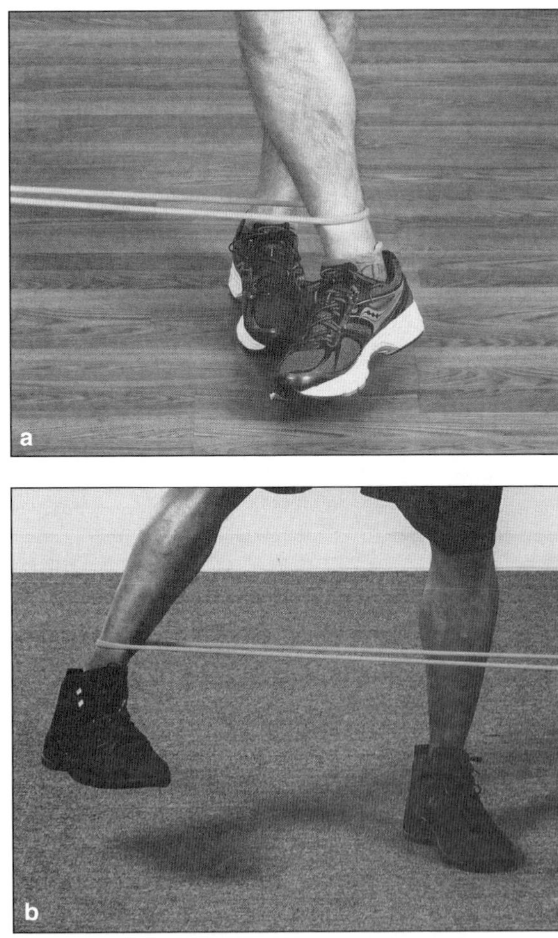

FIGURE 7.7 *(a)* Adduction with foot variation; *(b)* abduction with foot variation.

- These muscles are often worked in a gym environment using a machine where a person sits with the hips in flexion. We recommend using the bands with clients standing so the hip joint is in neutral, since many people have their hips in flexion for most of the day while sitting.
- Because adductor muscles are small and rarely included in workout sessions, start with the easiest band or no band at all to minimize risk for injury.

Strengthen the Shins

If clients are experiencing sore shins, here are three shin strengtheners they can do on their own. Caution clients not to do all the moves on the same day.

- *Heel walks*—During warm-ups, cool-downs, or anytime, walk around on the heels to strengthen shins. Start with just a few seconds and gradually build to about a minute at a time. This can be done daily and incorporated into classes.
- *Toe taps*—While sitting with the feet flat on the floor, lift the feet off the floor, keeping the heel down. Lower the feet down, flat on the floor. Do 8 to 12 reps, 1 to 3 sets. Do this daily.
- *Toe pulls*—Attach a resistance band around a sturdy piece of furniture or a railing. Sit on the floor with the left leg straight and the right one bent. Loop the band around the left foot. Flex the left foot, pulling the toes toward the shin and against the band (figure 7.8). Slowly release but only to neutral. Avoid pointing the toes so that the band stays in place. Do 1 to 3 sets, 8 to 12 reps, two or three days a week.

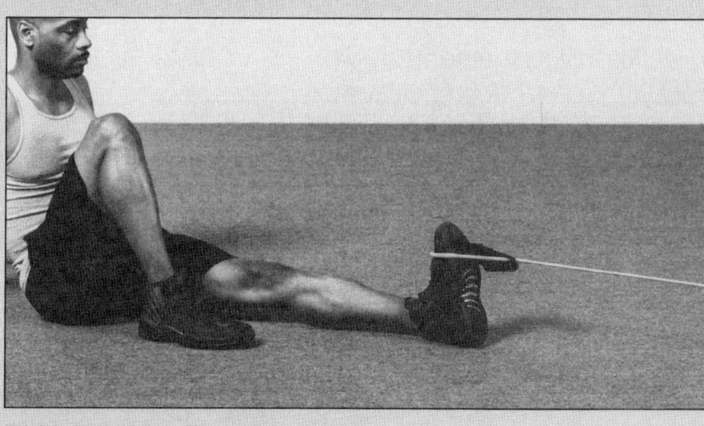

FIGURE 7.8 Toe pulls.

STANDING LEG ADDUCTION AND ABDUCTION *(continued)*

Cues That Work

- Stand tall.
- Breathe.
- Pull the navel toward the spine.
- Visualize pulling the weight-bearing leg toward the moving leg during adduction.
- Squeeze the shoulder blades together slightly to increase stability.

LAT PULL DOWNS

Muscles Targeted

Prime movers: latissimus dorsi

Synergists and stabilizers: trapezius, rhomboids, deltoids, biceps, triceps, flexors, serratus anterior

Equipment

Resistance band

BASIC LAT PULL-DOWN

1. Begin with the feet hip-width apart, holding the ends of the resistance band in each hand with the arms wide and overhead but slightly forward (figure 7.9*a*).
2. Exhale while pulling the hands away from each other and down, straightening the arms, until the band just touches a point about midway on the sternum (figure 7.9*b*).
3. Inhale while returning the arms to the overhead start position.
4. Do 8 to 12 repetitions.

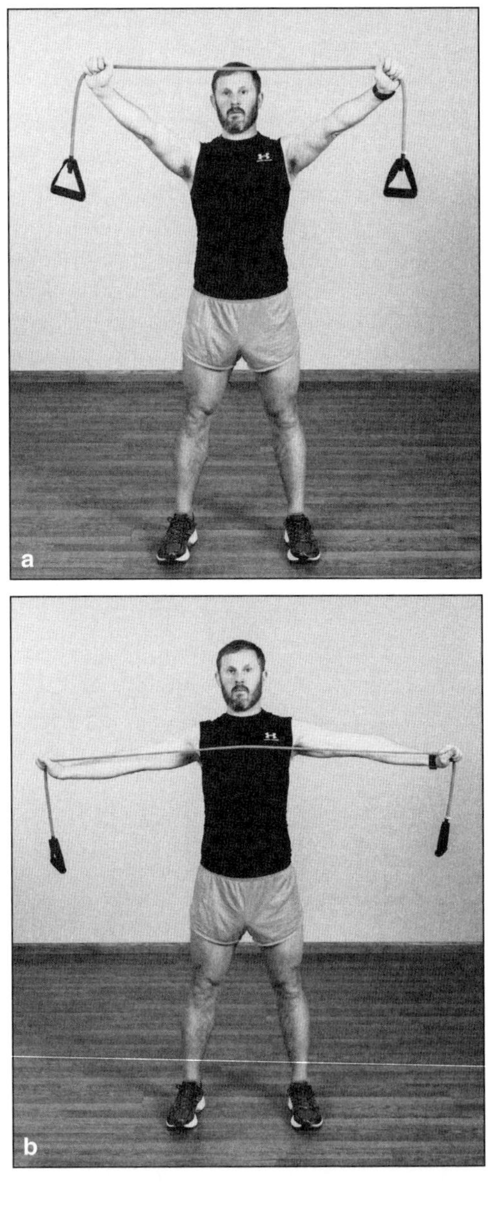

FIGURE 7.9 Basic lat pull-down: *(a)* start position and *(b)* down position.

Lat Pull-Down Variations

- Increase the resistance of the band to increase challenge.
- Change the count pace. Slow the inhalation or exhalation phases: Inhale for half the time of the exhale phase or inhale for double the time of the exhale phase.
- Hold the left hand in the start position and exhale while pulling down on the right side only, maintaining a straight right arm as it moves (figure 7.10). Inhale to return that right arm to the start position. Do 8 to 12 repetitions. Repeat holding the right hand steady and pull down on the left side only.

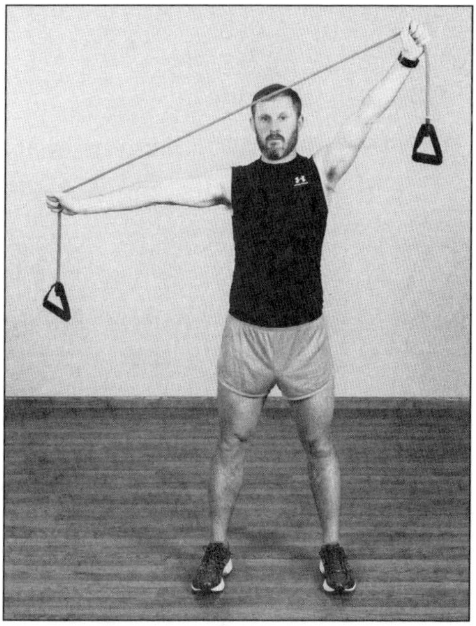

FIGURE 7.10 Single-arm lat pull-down variation.

Consider This

It's always helpful to know why you are recommending an exercise and relay that information to your clients. Here are a few tips to help your clients experience success.

- The muscles targeted by the lat pull-down are used for propulsive purposes as the arm moves back during the gait while walking. If these muscles are strong, your clients have more force to move the body forward. This is also a highly functional exercise to improve posture.
- We encourage doing this exercise standing because we tend to do enough sitting! Watch for the elbows bending as a sign that the band offers too much resistance.
- Check that the band always stays in front of the head. It should be visible when looking up with the eyes. People seem to think the band should be pulled down behind the neck, but this puts the shoulder at risk for serious injury.
- Stretching the band down enough to touch the breastbone is a cue that full range of motion through the shoulder has occurred. If you see people bending their elbows to pull the band down and then extending at the elbow to press their hands out the side, the band is too stiff, and they are putting themselves at risk for shoulder injury. Support the client in changing to a less-resistant band or moving their hands farther apart for more slack in the band and less resistance.
- It is tempting for people to hold their breath during this exercise. Advise when to inhale and when to exhale. Counting is encouraged at the exertion point to ensure they are exhaling.

Cues That Work

- Stand tall with the crown of head to the sky and the gaze to the horizon.
- Maintain straight, but not locked, elbows as the arms pull away from each other.
- Squeeze the shoulder blades toward each other.
- Exhale on the exertion.
- Return to the start position when the band touches the breastbone.
- Inhale to return.

STANDING ROW

Muscles Targeted

Prime movers: latissimus dorsi, rhomboids

Synergists and stabilizers: trapezius, rotator cuff, teres major, teres minor, forearm muscles, pectoralis major

Equipment

Resistance band; sturdy object to use as an anchor

BASIC STANDING ROW

1. With the band attached to a fixed point at waist level, place the feet in a position that mimics the walking stance, with the left foot ahead and the right foot behind. Hold the band in the right hand in a handshake position (figure 7.11*a*).
2. Exhale while bending the elbow and pulling the band back to the hip bone or farther. Keep the elbow pointing behind and close to the body, not pointing out to the side (figure 7.11*b*).

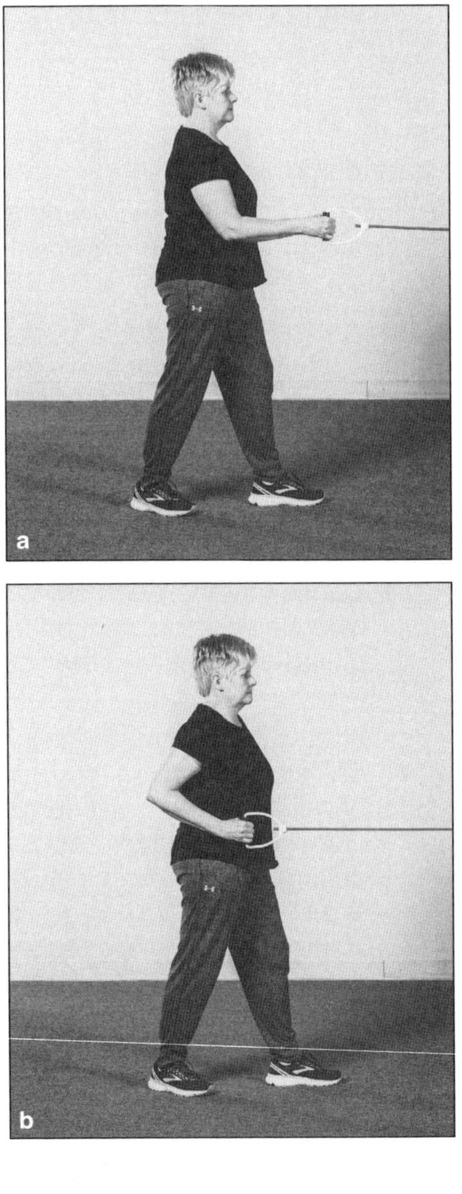

FIGURE 7.11 Basic standing row: *(a)* start position and *(b)* pull position.

3. Inhale while extending the arm to the starting position.
4. Do 8 to 12 repetitions.
5. Switch legs and repeat with the left hand holding the band.

Standing Row Variations

- Increase the resistance of the band to make it more challenging.
- Variations in hand position can maintain interest and recruit slightly different muscle fibers. For example, externally rotate the forearm so that the palm faces sky, or internally rotate it so that the palm faces the ground.
- Stand on one leg only, the leg opposite to the hand that is holding the band. This recruits the muscles of the core and the stabilizing muscles of the weight-bearing leg.

Consider This

The standing row is helpful for walkers because the motion is what we encourage in progressions 1 and 3 of the walking technique—bent arms and driving the arm back. Here are things to consider to ensure success.

- *Specificity*—The standing row exercise targets muscles of the upper back and posterior shoulder muscles, including the latissimus dorsi and the rhomboids, in a way that is more specific than the lat pull-down by more directly mimicking the motion of the arms while walking.
- *Get the right challenge*—Help them find a resistance band that allows them to bring the hand back at least as far as the hip bone. If they can't pull the hand back to the hip, they need lighter resistance. Sometimes standing closer to the anchor point of the band will reduce resistance and allow the hand to meet the hip or adjusting the hand placement on the band so that there is more slack.
- *Staying upright*—If stability is an issue when the feet are staggered, ensure that their feet are positioned hip-width apart in this staggered position.

Cues That Work

- Stand tall.
- Look to the horizon.
- Squeeze the shoulder blades toward the middle of the back.
- Pull the navel toward the spine for greater stability.
- Exhale on the exertion.
- Count on the exertion!
- Inhale to return.

SIDE PLANK

Muscles Targeted

Prime movers: transversus abdominis, rectus abdominis, internal and external obliques, quadratus lumborum, gluteus medius and minimus

Synergists and stabilizers: gluteus maximus, quadriceps, hamstrings

Equipment Needed

Elevated surface

ELEVATED SIDE PLANK

1. Stand with the right side of the body facing an elevated, level surface, such as a picnic table or bench.
2. Place the right forearm on the elevated surface, and extend the legs so that the body is in a straight line, with the side of the right foot on the ground in line with the right hip, shoulder, and ear. Place the left leg slightly behind the right foot on the ground for stability. Shoulders should be stacked over the elbow (figure 7.12).
3. Maintain the position with isometric muscle contraction for 8 to 12 breath cycles.
4. Switch sides and repeat.

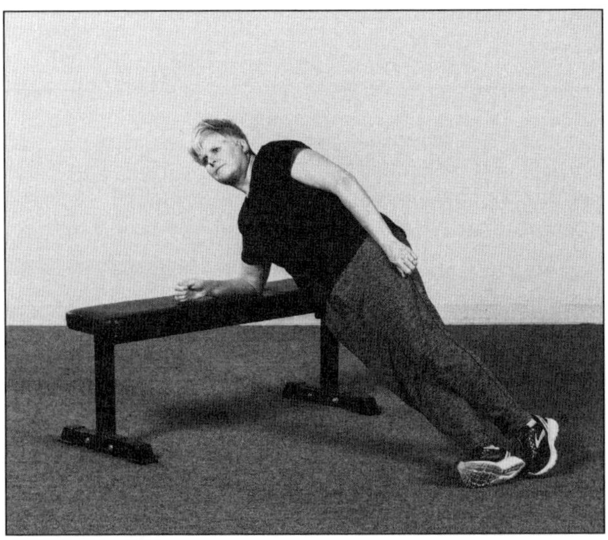

FIGURE 7.12 Elevated side plank.

SIDE PLANK WITH STACKED FEET

1. Stand with the right side of the body facing an elevated, level surface, such as a picnic table or bench.
2. Place the right forearm on the elevated surface, and extend the legs so that the body is in a straight line, with the side of the right foot on the ground in line with the right hip, shoulder, and ear. Place the left leg and foot on top of the right leg and foot (figure 7.13). Shoulders should be stacked over the elbow.
3. Maintain the position with isometric muscle contraction for 8 to 12 breath cycles.
4. Switch sides and repeat.

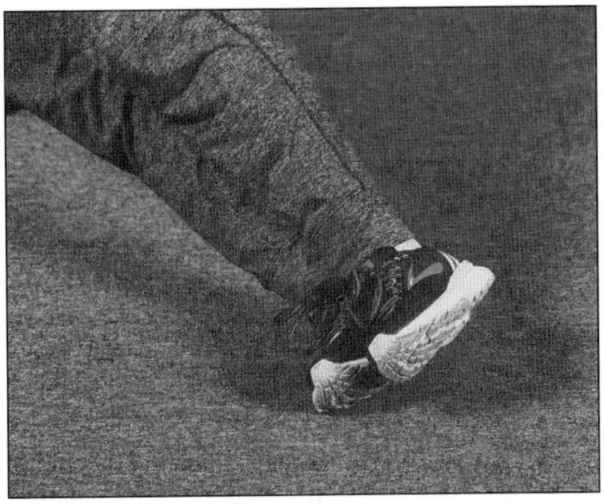

FIGURE 7.13 Side plank with stacked. feet

SIDE PLANK WITH HIP DROP AND RAISE

1. Stand with the right side of the body facing an elevated, level surface, such as a picnic table or bench.
2. Place the right forearm on the elevated surface, and extend the legs so that the body is in a straight line, with the side of the right foot on the ground in line with the right hip, shoulder, and ear. Place the left leg slightly behind the right foot on the ground. Shoulders should be stacked over the elbow.
3. Inhale while lowering the right hip toward the ground (figure 7.14).
4. Exhale while contracting the right side of the waist to lift the right hip and return to the starting position.
5. Do 8 to 12 repetitions.
6. Repeat on the other side.

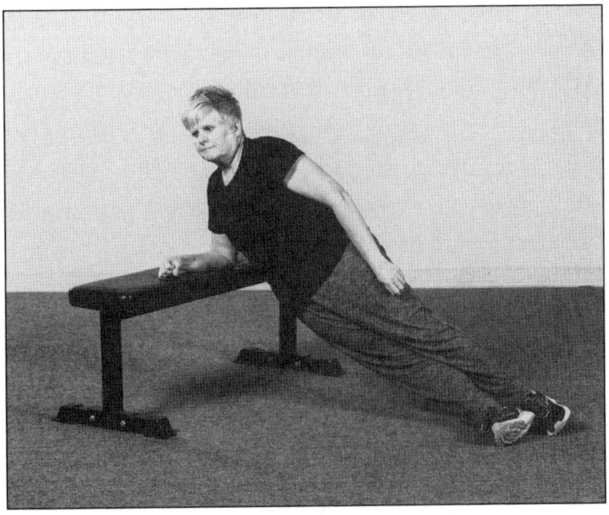

FIGURE 7.14 Side plank with hip drop.

Consider This

Side planks offer a fantastic opportunity to recruit the spine-stabilizing muscles of the abdominals, especially the external and internal obliques, transversus abdominis, and quadratus lumborum. In addition to maintaining spinal stability, these muscles facilitate a powerful walking gait, particularly when walkers add hip rotation (see Progression 4 in chapter 4).

- *Alignment matters*—Look for the top hip to be stacked over the bottom hip. Make sure the head is pulled back so that ear is in line with the ankles, hips, and shoulders.
- *Set up for success*—Begin clients on an easy progression to ensure that they learn good form. The higher the elevation, the easier it is, so find places where this can be taught using different elevations. If stairs are available, this is probably the best way to progress with the side plank for two reasons: The positioning at a higher stair is easier for stability and muscle contraction, and the upper arm can be supported by the riser of the stair when balancing on the forearm. Picnic tables and benches are good alternatives if there are no stairs. You can even teach side planks against trees.
- *Progress gradually*—Start with the feet wide for stability (foot of the top leg placed behind the foot of the bottom leg to keep the top hip stacked over the bottom hip) and progress to stacked feet.
- *Find what works*—Doing the side plank from the forearm is easier for most people than balancing on the hand and straight arm. Also, balancing on the forearm makes the abdominal challenge more difficult than balancing on the hand with a straight arm. Give people time to experiment with both.

Cues That Work

- Pull the head back for spinal alignment.
- Breathe. (Possibly advise when to inhale and when to exhale.)
- Pull the navel toward the spine.
- Squeeze the shoulder blades together slightly.
- Release the hip toward ground while keeping the body in alignment (for the hip drop).
- Engage the muscles at the waist on the side facing toward the ground to return to the start position (for the hip drop).
- Minimize shoulder movement so that the work is happening at the waist (for the hip drop).
- Pain in the shoulder joint? Engage navel to spine and step out to re-align the shoulder over the elbow.

PUSH-UPS

Muscles Targeted

Prime movers: pectoralis major, anterior deltoids, triceps brachii

Additional muscles targeted: triceps (narrow push-up exercise)

Synergists and stabilizers: rectus abdominis, transverse abdominis, quadriceps, pectoralis minor

Equipment Needed

Elevated surface

BASIC PUSH-UP

1. Place the hands wider than shoulder-width apart on an elevated railing or picnic table. Step back with both feet far enough that the body is a straight line from heels to ears. Heels should be off the ground, balancing on the balls of the feet and toes.
2. Inhale while bending the elbows and lowering the sternum toward the railing or table, ensuring the elbows line up over the wrists (figure 7.15).
3. Exhale while straightening the arms to push the chest away from the railing or table.
4. Do 8 to 12 repetitions.

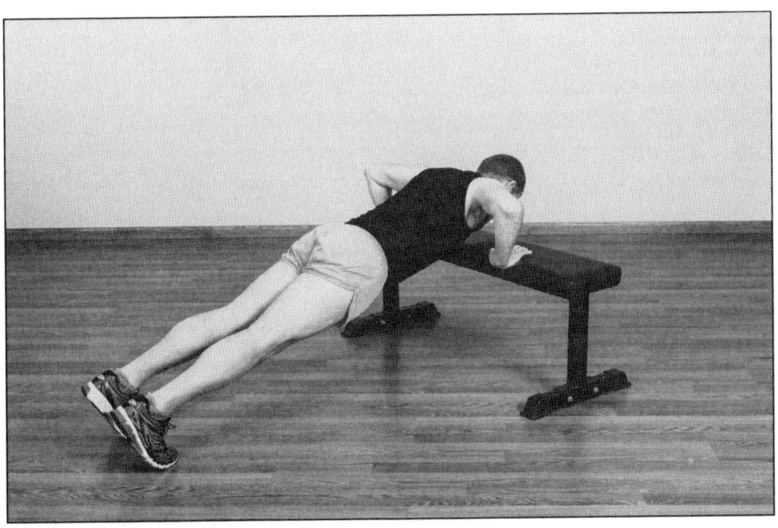

FIGURE 7.15 Basic push-up.

SINGLE-LEG PUSH-UP

1. Place the hands wider than shoulder-width apart on an elevated railing or picnic table. Step back with both feet far enough that the body is a straight line from heels to ears. Lift one foot off the ground.
2. Inhale while bending the elbows and lowering the sternum toward the railing or table, ensuring the elbows line up over the wrists (figure 7.16).
3. Exhale while straightening the arms to push the chest away from the railing or table.
4. Do 4 to 6 repetitions.
5. Repeat on the other leg.

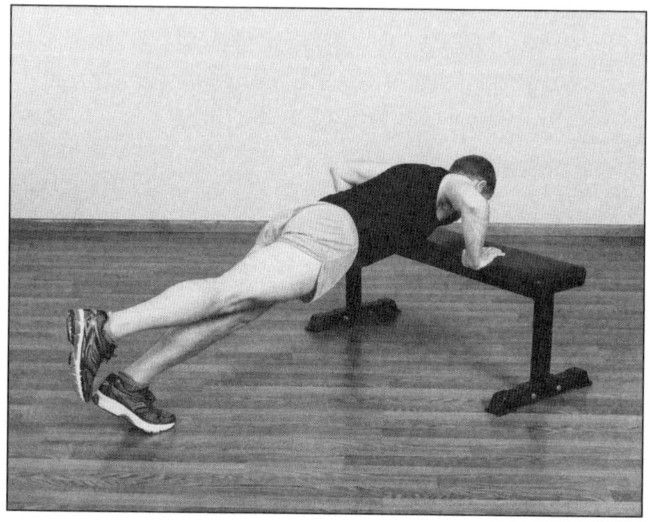

FIGURE 7.16 Single-leg push-up.

NARROW PUSH-UP

1. Place the hands in line with the shoulders on an elevated railing or picnic table. Step back with both feet far enough that the body is a straight line from heels to ears.
2. Inhale while bending the elbows, hugging them in close to the sides of the body, and lower the sternum toward the railing or table, maintaining contraction of the shoulder blades so the elbows are pulling toward each other (figure 7.17).
3. Exhale while straightening the arms to push chest away from the railing or table.
4. Do 8 to 12 repetitions.

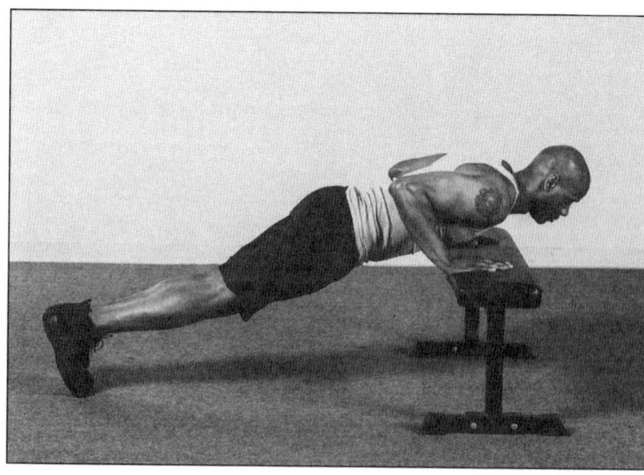

FIGURE 7.17 Narrow push-up.

Consider This

Give your clients a sense of power when doing push-ups well. There are many things to watch for and tips to offer for this total-body exercise.

- *Why we do it*—The push-up, although it works the chest muscles and we typically recommend a focus on muscles of the posterior chain, is a whole-body exercise that also activates the abdominals and leg muscles as stabilizers. The straight spine position encourages good posture.
- *Use your environment*—Done easily outdoors using railings, picnic tables, and even trees, the push-up works well in all seasons.
- *Watch for hips that are out of alignment with the spine*—People may drop them too low toward the ground or raise them too high toward the sky.
- *Encouragement proper breathing*—Inhale on lowering into the push-up and exhale on exertion as they straighten the arms.
- *Set up for success*—Encourage people to start at the highest height possible for hand placement. If more than 12 repetitions are readily accessible at this height, suggest they move to a lower elevation for a greater challenge.

Cues That Work

- Wide hands!
- Reach the sternum toward the railing or bench, inhaling as you reach.
- Imagine a straight line from the heels to the crown of the head.
- Balance on the balls and toes of your feet; heels off the ground.
- Exhale on the exertion.
- Pull the navel toward the spine.
- Keep the navel pulled in as you step in to exit from the exercise.
- Elbows hugged in (for the narrow push-up).

Home Workout Ideas

Here are a couple of our favorite exercises that are easier done at home than in an outdoor class. Not everyone likes to get close to the ground, and it's not that easy to bring a stability ball for everyone. Both exercises (bridge and plank) emphasize strengthening the muscles that lie between the hips and the shoulders. That's the core! A strong core works for life and for walking.

BRIDGE

Muscles Targeted

Prime movers: gluteus maximus, hamstrings

Synergists and stabilizers: transversus abdominis, gluteus medius and minimus, adductor group

Equipment Needed

Stability ball

DYNAMIC BRIDGE

1. Lie on the back, the knees bent and feet flat on the floor, hip-width apart, and at a comfortable distance from the hips. Extend the arms at the sides, palms down.
2. Inhale while pressing the feet into the floor and lifting the hips off floor toward the ceiling until the body forms a straight line from shoulders to knees (figure 7.18).
3. Exhale while lowering the hips a few inches toward floor.
4. Lift and lower 8 to 12 repetitions.

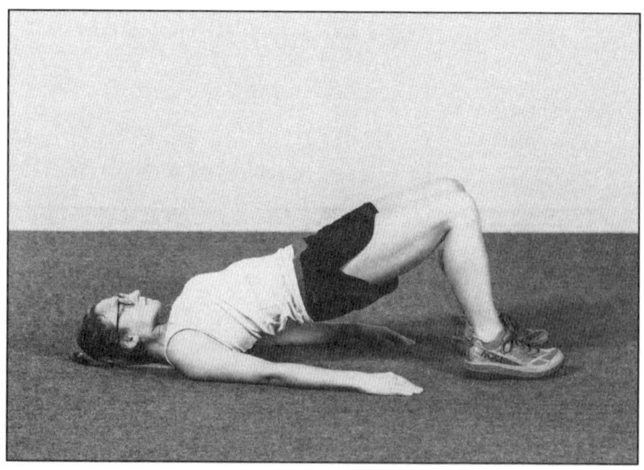

FIGURE 7.18 Dynamic bridge.

STATIC BRIDGE WITH ALTERNATING KNEE EXTENSION

1. Lie on the back, knees bent, feet flat on the floor hip-width apart, and at a comfortable distance from the hips. Extend the arms at the sides. Put the palms down.
2. Inhale while pressing the feet into the floor and lifting the hips off floor toward the ceiling until the body forms a straight line from shoulders to knees.
3. Inhale while lifting the right foot off the floor, keeping the leg bent.
4. Exhale while straightening that leg (figure 7.19).
5. Inhale while bending the knee in that elevated position.
6. Exhale while lowering the right foot to the floor.
7. Repeat with left leg.
8. Alternate legs for 8 to 12 repetitions with each leg while holding the bridge position.

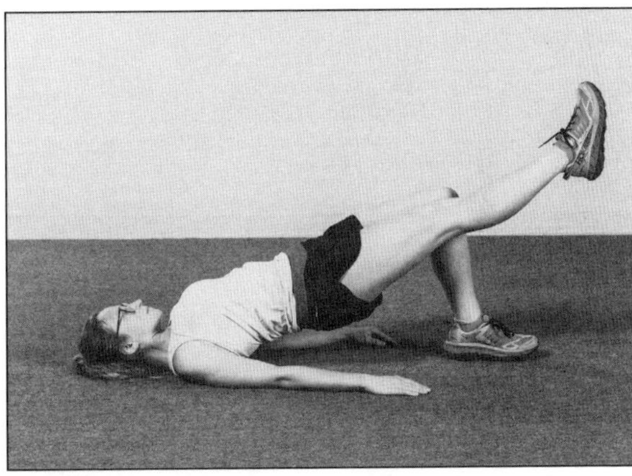

FIGURE 7.19 Static bridge with alternating knee extension.

BRIDGE USING A STABILITY BALL

1. Lie on the back, legs straight and heels resting on a stability ball. Extend the arms along the sides.
2. Inhale while lifting the hips off the floor into a straight-leg bridge position (figure 7.20*a*).
3. Exhale while bending the knees and pulling the ball toward hips with feet (figure 7.20*b*).
4. Inhale while straightening the legs.
5. Repeat flexion and extension of knee joint for 8 to 12 repetitions.
6. Exhale while slowly lowering the body to rest on the floor.

BRIDGE USING A STABILITY BALL *(continued)*

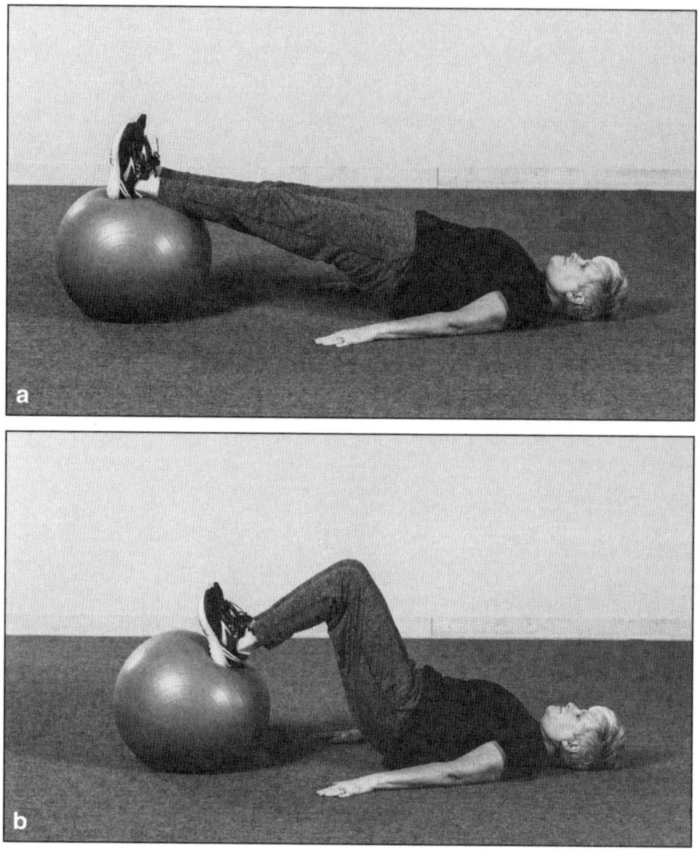

FIGURE 7.20 Bridge using a stability ball: *(a)* with legs extended and *(b)* with ball pulled toward hips.

Consider This

Bridge exercises strengthen the posterior chain muscles and stretch the anterior chain muscles to counteract the constant flexion of the spine many people experience in daily life. Here are things to consider to ensure clients maximize success.

- Watch for the knees collapsing toward each other in bridge. A common trick used by yoga instructors is to place a yoga block between the inner thighs. Rolled up towels, soccer balls, or basketballs would work too.
- Stability balls are easier to use if they are slightly deflated.

Cues That Work

- Walk the shoulders away from the ears before lifting the hips.
- Actively press the feet into the floor as the hips lift.
- Ensure that the knees remain hip-width apart.
- Breathe.
- Lower the hips to the floor while maintaining a lordotic curve in the low back.

PLANK

Muscles Targeted

Prime movers: rectus abdominis, transversus abdominis

Additional muscles targeted: oblique abdominals (static plank with waist rotation)

Synergists and stabilizers: oblique abdominals, hip flexor group, quadriceps group, pectoralis major, serratus anterior

Equipment Needed

Stability ball

STATIC PLANK

1. Begin facedown on the floor. Place the elbows under the shoulders so that forearms rest on the floor.
2. Tuck the toes and push into the hands and forearms while inhaling to lift the body off the floor, hips in line with the shoulders and head (figure 7.21). Pull the navel toward the spine while maintaining this position for 8 to 10 breath cycles.
3. Exhale while lowering the knees and bringing the belly to the ground.

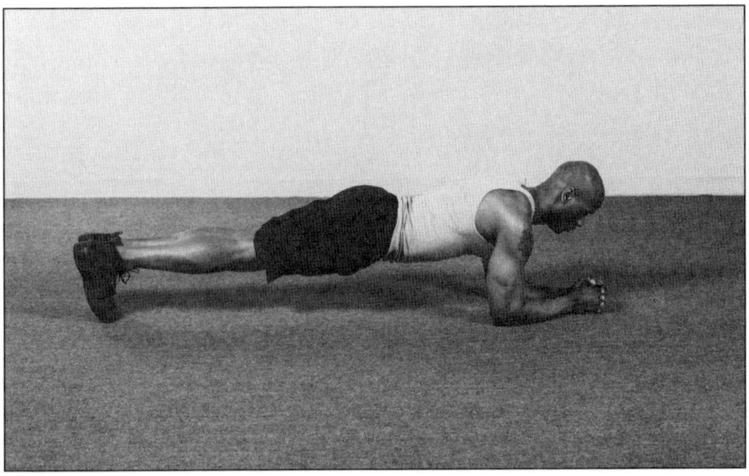

FIGURE 7.21 Static plank.

STATIC PLANK WITH WAIST ROTATION

1. Begin facedown on the floor. Place the elbows under the shoulders so that forearms rest on the floor.
2. Tuck the toes and push into the hands and forearms while inhaling to lift the body off the floor, hips in line with the shoulders and head. Exhale while pulling the navel toward the spine.
3. Inhale while rotating the torso at the waist, lowering the right hip toward the floor without touching the floor (figure 7.22).
4. Exhale while returning the right hip to neutral.
5. Inhale while rotating the torso at the waist, lowering the left hip toward the floor without touching the floor.
6. Exhale while returning the left hip to neutral.
7. Do 8 to 12 of these hip dips on each side.
8. Exhale while lowering the knees and belly to the ground.

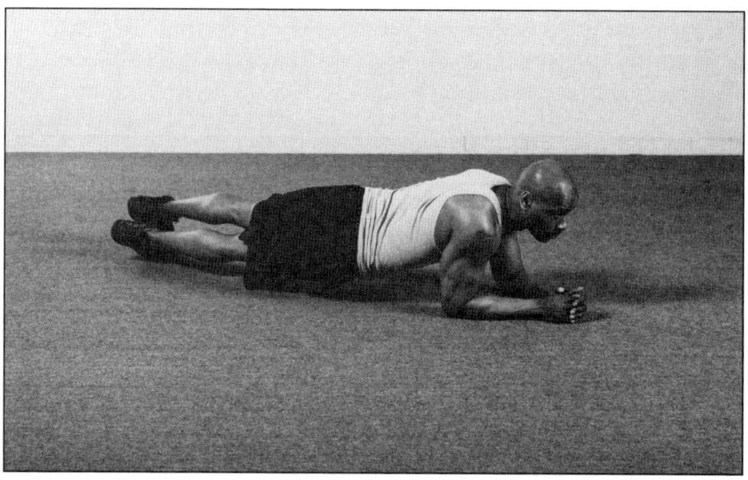

FIGURE 7.22 Static plank with waist rotation.

PLANK USING A STABILITY BALL

1. Kneeling on the floor, place the bent elbows and forearms on a stability ball.
2. Inhale while stepping back with one foot and then the other to arrive in the plank position on top of the stability ball (figure 7.23*a*).
3. Inhale while pulling the navel to the spine and releasing the elbows forward an inch or two (figure 7.23*b*).
4. Exhale while pulling the navel toward spine and pulling the forearms back to the starting position.
5. Do this forearm slide back and forth 8 to 12 repetitions.

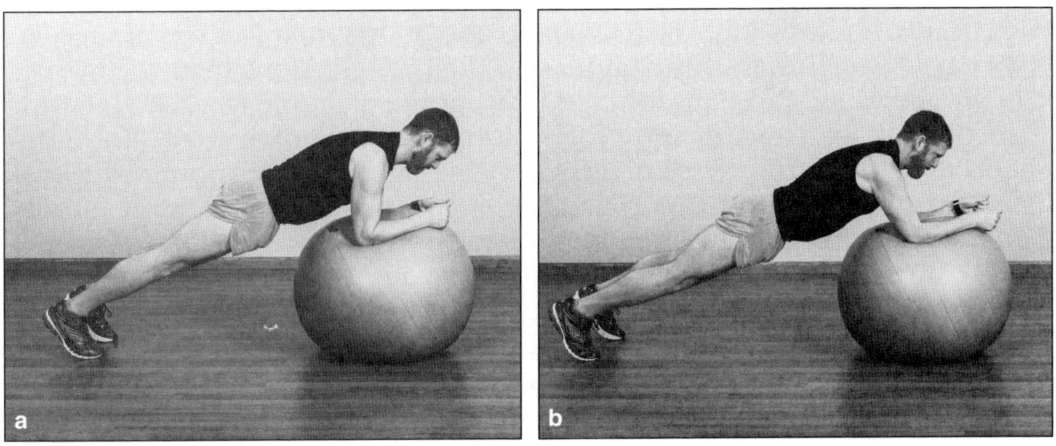

FIGURE 7.23 Plank using a stability ball.

Consider This

It is difficult to fatigue the abdominal muscles, so doing planks frequently at home is great advice for your clients. Here are tips to make it work for them.

- Starting a plank from an elevation higher than the floor sets people up for success. Suggest placing forearms on a third or fourth stair, chair, or other firm surface. As they feel stronger, they can move to a lower position.
- Check in at the hips. The hip position is often either too high or too low. If possible, demonstrate these two misalignments followed by the correct position. If the hips are too low, it can strain the back. They should never feel pain in the low back. If the hips are too high, the abdominals are not challenged.
- Stability balls are easier to use if they are slightly deflated.
- Avoid hunching the shoulders by pulling the shoulders away from the ears, creating space between the shoulders and ears.

Cues That Work

- Inhale to lift the hips and belly.
- Pull the forearms toward feet to engage the abs isometrically (this also keeps shoulders from being hunched). Actively press the feet into the floor as the hips lift.
- Keep the crown of the head in line with the heels.
- If it's too easy, the hips are probably too high.
- Breathe.

Introducing strength exercises empowers your walkers to experience the myriad benefits that we know result from improved muscle strength. And, as a bonus, it makes them faster walkers and boosts their feelings of success. The seven exercises in this chapter and their progressions work well when incorporated into an outdoor class. Try adding a couple to each workout. The two indoor exercises and progressions give additional attention to the abdominals, muscles that are difficult to fatigue and contribute to spinal stability and well-being. Coach and encourage clients to do strength "homework." Just a few exercises can be integrated into a daily routine as clients are waiting for dinner to cook in the oven, during a commercial break if they are watching television, or as part of an after-dinner routine. As we move into part IV, you'll discover ways to create walking classes that work for the many people who love to walk and will come to your classes to enjoy a challenging and structured walking workout.

References

1. Clark, T.C., Norris, T., and Schiller, J.S. 2017. Early Release of Selected Estimates Based on Data From the 2016 National Health Interview Survey. National Center for Health Statistics. www.cdc.gov/nchs/data/nhis/earlyrelease/earlyrelease201705.pdf.
2. Willen, C., Sunnerhagen, K.S., Ekman, C., and Grimby, G. 2004. "How Is Walking Speed Related to Muscle Strength? A Study of Healthy Persons and Persons With Late Effects of Polio." *Archives of Physical Medicine and Rehabilitation* 85 (12): 1923-28. www.archives-pmr.org/article/S0003-9993(04)00188-1/fulltext.
3. Van Abbema, R., DeGreef, M., Craje, C., Krijnen, W., Hobbelen, H., and Van Der Schans, C. 2015. "What Type or Combination of Exercise Can Improve Preferred Gait Speed in Older Adults? A Meta-Analysis." *BMC Geriatrics* 15: 72-87. www.ncbi.nlm.nih.gov/pmc/articles/PMC4488060/pdf/12877_2015_Article_61.pdf.
4. Seguin, R.A., Eldridge, G., Lynch, W., and Paul, L.C. 2013. "Strength Training Improves Body Image and Physical Activity Behaviors Among Midlife and Older Rural Women." *Journal of Extension* 51 (4): 1-14. www.joe.org/joe/2013august/pdf/JOE_v51_4a2.pdf.
5. Martin Ginis, K.A., Eng, J.J., Arbour, K.P., Hartman, J.W., and Phillips, S.M. 2005. "Mind Over Muscle? Sex Differences in the Relationship Between Body Image Change and Subjective and Objective Physical Changes Following a 12-Week Strength Training Program." *Body Image* 2 (4): 363-72. www.ncbi.nlm.nih.gov/pubmed/18089201.

PART IV

ENHANCE THE EXPERIENCE

8

Ensure Comfort and Safety

Contentment, well-being, mental health, and physical health are all benefits of a daily walk. These benefits are accessible to most people as part of daily physical activity—walking to complete errands, taking stairs instead of escalators or elevators, walking to work, and walking meetings. In order to conduct a successful walking program, the accessibility of walking cannot be taken for granted. There are barriers to walking, and the better they are addressed, the more likely people will commit to your walking program.

In this chapter, we'll talk about how to make walking programs enticing and sustainable for as many people as possible. We'll cover what to wear, venue safety issues, and how to navigate several weather conditions.

Comfort Is Key

One of the reasons walking is popular is because it doesn't require any special clothing or gear. We can walk in whatever we're wearing. Put on a pair of sneakers, and we can walk home from the office, take a walk to meet a friend, or pick up a child from school. This ease appeals to many people when they consider joining a walking program, so it's a bit of a balancing act when advising walkers on apparel—and another reason to understand your audience. If they are already avid walkers who want to take walking to the next level, discussions on technical gear are likely to inspire and motivate them. For those just trying to make walking a habit, it may discourage them. If they think that they have to worry about what they are wearing, it creates another obstacle, giving them one more excuse for staying home. For them, the idea of not having to change clothes to go for a walk may be more likely to get them going. So, when discussing apparel, emphasize that it is a personal preference, not a requirement.

The key message to relay about sport-specific technical clothing is that it improves performance by increasing comfort. For example, the right clothing can prevent one of the biggest walking discomforts: skin chafing. Skin-to-skin contact, such as under the arms and between the thighs, may lead to intense chafing that can cause breakage of the skin.

In addition, research has shown that wearing specialty clothes for exercise creates a mindset of empowerment, commitment, self-efficacy, and excellence. When avid walkers were surveyed, 45 percent of them said that clothing and gear helped keep them motivated [1]. Let's look at what you and your participants might need or want, from bottom to top, when it comes to apparel.

Feet

When our feet are happy while we walk, the chances are the rest of the body will feel pretty good, too. Despite barefoot movement trends in running and walking, we still think wearing shoes is the safer route and the way to get improved performance out of the body during workouts.

Shoes

Something as simple as feeling that a special pair of shoes are necessary to start walking can be a barrier to getting active. Everyone has favorite shoes, and many of them will be perfectly good for a walking workout. The shoes your clients currently wear to go out for a stroll are the shoes to use when trying the first walking workout. Having said that, as your clients begin to walk faster and go farther, they may notice that their shoes need to change—usually identified by the fact that improvements to gait and speed are plateauing. They might also notice heat building up in the heel area, which is often a sign to move to a shoe with a slightly lower heel and slightly less cushioning. But that doesn't mean clients have to invest in the most expensive pair. When Scottish researchers [2] tested running shoes that cost $80 to $150, they found that the lower-priced shoes performed just as well as the higher-priced ones. Here are suggestions for the shoe characteristics that might improve walking, especially for those who want walking to be their main form of aerobic exercise.

Training Shoes Versus Running Shoes. Looking at a wall of dozens of shoes in a store can be overwhelming. There are sport-specific athletic shoes for just about every type of activity, from basketball and tennis to cycling and even yoga. Cross-trainers are a popular style that sound like they would be good for walking, but they are not the best choice. These shoes are typically designed with lateral support for workouts that incorporate side-to-side movement, such as aerobics classes, CrossFit, and other workouts that feature lateral movements. Surprisingly, running shoes are the best option for walking. They are designed for forward and back movement and tend to feature more cushioning in the heel, which many walkers like. While there are shoes designed specifically for walkers (figure 8.1), many are heavy and stiff, and we have found that most of our clients prefer running styles—us too! More than 10 years ago, when a trend toward light, minimalist running shoes with low heel profiles and thin soles became popular for runners, the power walker benefited in ways that we will soon discuss.

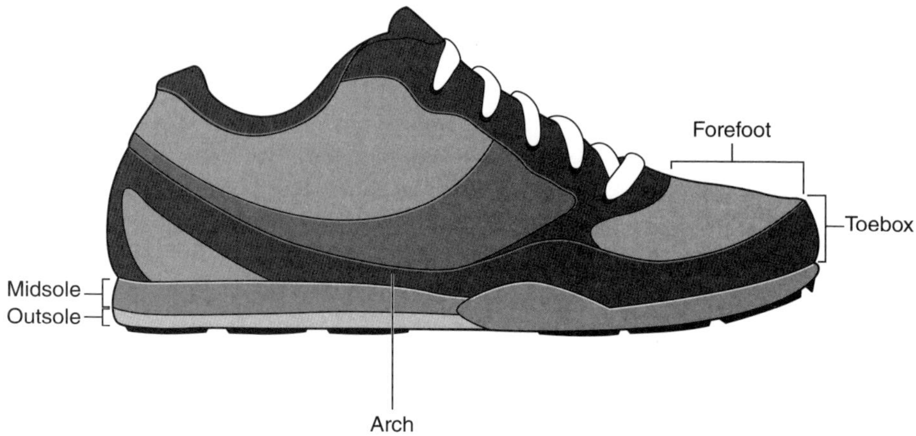

FIGURE 8.1 Anatomy of a walking shoe: heel, forefoot, arch, sole, toebox.

To help navigate all the choices, we recommend shopping at a specialty running store. Although they may not have an expertise in walking, they will have experience with the various shoes on the market, and they will understand what shoes suit each individual because different body types, gaits, and foot movement have different shoe requirements. Here are tips to share with your clients to help ensure a successful purchase:

- Shop late in the day when feet are usually at their largest from standing and other activity throughout the day.
- Bring a pair of well-used walking shoes so that the salesperson can see the wear pattern on the tread. This identifies foot movement as either neutral, pronating, or supinating, which helps them suggest a suitable shoe. Feet that overpronate (foot rolls toward midline) or oversupinate (foot rolls to outer edges of foot) will need shoes with appropriate support to neutralize the gait.
- Remember socks. They can affect the fit of a shoe. While trying on shoes, wear the socks that will be worn while walking. (See advice on selecting socks later in this chapter.)
- Test the shoes before purchase. Specialty stores understand the need for this, so they are more likely to let people go outside or provide a treadmill for a test walk. At the very least, they'll let people take a few laps around the inside of the store. Try on several brands, even wearing a different one on each foot, for comparison. If there is any rubbing, discomfort, or hot spots, try another pair. The right shoe will feel good right away, and no "breaking in" is necessary.

Heel Cushioning. Heel cushioning in running shoes can create a difference in height between the forefoot and the heel that is described as the heel-to-toe drop or offset (figure 8.2). Note that it is possible to have cushioning built into a shoe at both heel and forefoot (see figure 8.1), resulting in no offset (8.2c). Shoes with a lot of cushioning at the heel will typically have a high heel-to-toe drop (8.2b); those with less cushioning will have a lower heel-to-toe drop (8.2a). While the extra cushioning can feel good when walking, there are reasons why some walkers may want to move toward a less cushioned shoe as they become more proficient with power walking. Excess cushioning limits the range of motion around the ankle for the heel-to-toe roll. Imagine how difficult it is to walk quickly wearing high-heeled dress shoes. This can happen with running shoes that have a high heel-to-toe drop, though in a less dramatic way. Also, when the heel strikes the ground in a shoe that is heavily cushioned at the heel, there will be energy lost into the foam and some shearing action through the foam. This means the body has less energy and power during the roll from heel strike to toe push-off. Think of race cars or road bicycles that have thinner tires than regular cars or mountain bikes. With these types of low-profile tires, the engine power of the car or the pedal work on the bicycle goes more directly into pushing the car or bicycle along the road rather than into the rubber of thicker tires to improve speed and performance. Similarly, thinner soles at the heel of running shoes (often referred to as a low heel profile) would be chosen to improve walking speed and performance. A change to a thinner-sole shoe should be done gradually so the body can adjust without injury. Still, for some walkers, extra heel cushioning will always be their preferred shoe construction.

Understanding that shoes with lower heel profiles and thinner soles will allow walkers to increase speed and improve performance, good coaches will monitor the walking technique of their clients. As they are able to shorten stride lengths in front of the body, reducing impact at the heel strike, they may be ready to try shoes that have a lower heel-to-toe drop and less cushioning.

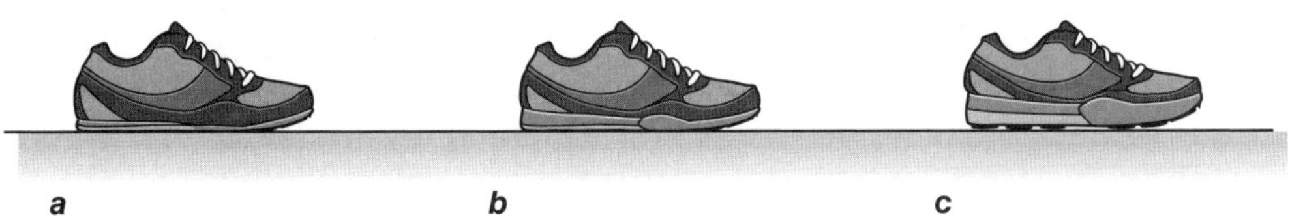

FIGURE 8.2 Example of thin sole, low offset (*a*). Example of thin sole, high offset (*b*). Example of thick sole, no offset (*c*).

Forefoot. In addition to the cushioning under the heel of running shoes, there is cushioning under the forefoot (metatarsal area; see figure 8.1). At the same time, this area tends to be fairly stiff in many shoe models because it improves running performance. Walking, however, needs more flexibility so that the forefoot can move easily through its entire range of motion to facilitate the toe push-off. Again, new walkers may be more comfortable in shoes with a well-cushioned and stiff forefoot because it is what they are used to wearing. As walking performance improves, walkers could be encouraged to try shoes with less cushioning and less stiffness in the forefoot to allow a strong toe push-off. Always take care to make any changes to shoes carefully and incrementally because these changes may affect gait and spinal alignment, increasing the possibility of discomfort and injury.

One final note about the front of walking shoes. Walkers should go up half a size from their regular shoes. This leaves room in the toe box area (see figure 8.1) for any swelling that is normal during walking workouts.

Replacing Shoes. Over time, shoe materials break down, making them less supportive. This deterioration is not always visible, so it is recommended that shoes be replaced at least every 300 to 500 miles. For example, someone who averages a 15-minute-per-mile pace and walks 3 hours a week would need to replace shoes every 6 to 9 months. Heavier walkers or those who notice the soles wearing down quickly or unevenly should replace them on the lower end of the range. Another indicator that it is time to replace shoes is if a walker notices any discomfort in the hips, knees, or feet. Although the exact cause is not easily discernible, it could be that the shoes are deteriorating and no longer absorbing shock or supporting gait.

Socks.

That thin sliver of material wrapping our feet inside our shoes can be the unsung hero for happy feet. Of course, the shoe itself is extremely important, but socks can have a dramatic effect on the walking workout experience. The feet need to stay as cool and dry as possible to avoid chafing and blistering while walking. Synthetic fabric that allows sweat to be pulled away from the skin is best. Socks with any cotton content will absorb moisture from the feet and may bunch in the shoe, causing blisters. When purchasing shoes, encourage clients to try them on with the socks they will wear during walking workouts because the thickness of socks can affect the fit and size of the shoe needed. Thicker socks may crowd the feet, causing blisters. Conversely, thinner socks may leave room for the foot to slide around in the shoe, also causing blisters. If clients wear socks when trying on shoes, they can find the right shoe in the right size to prevent this, and their socks and shoes will work together well.

In winter, the feet may not sweat as much as at other times of the year and may even get cold. Thicker socks may keep feet warm, although clients will need to consider the possibility that the extra thickness might restrict the feet in such a way that actually makes them colder. Alternatively, they may find that a sock of the same thickness as a synthetic sock but made of merino wool helps. Wool tends to keep us warm even when wet. In extreme cold, below 14 degrees F (-10 degrees C), we have used neoprene toe caps placed over socks. The neoprene is quite thin but, again, may affect the fit of the shoe in the same way that thick socks do.

Whether your clients go with thicker or thinner socks is a personal preference. We experience less heat build-up and fewer blisters with thin socks. However, many others prefer thicker socks with more cushioning. Whatever type of sock is worn when trying on and purchasing shoes, encourage clients to have at least two to three pairs of those socks available to wear with their walking shoes.

The other consideration is the style of sock, such as a low rise that comes just above the top of the shoe and below the ankle or socks that cover the ankle. This choice is also about personal preference. Another popular style is the compression sock that covers the lower leg and applies increased pressure. Unless clients have a condition that requires wearing compression socks and a doctor has recommended doing so, there is little evidence that performance will improve if they wear them while walking. Also, they can be costly.

Seasonal Considerations.

Typically, we wear the same shoes all year around, but there are winter options that walkers may want to consider. Shoes made of GoreTex help keep feet dry. Shoes with windproof material (no mesh or a tighter

Treat Your Feet

We walk all over them every day and usually don't pay them any attention until they start to hurt. Don't wait until pain strikes to give feet a little attention. The small muscles in the toes work to maintain balance and roll feet through their full range of motion, keeping them strong and flexible is important. Strong foot and ankle muscles also enhance mobility. Here are easy exercises for both you and your clients to keep feet healthy and happy. Aim to do these moves three or four times a week.

- *Alphabet.* Sitting on a high stool or counter so the legs are hanging, use the right foot to write the alphabet in the air. The writing motions should come from the ankle; think of the toes as the point of a pencil. Repeat with the left foot.
- *Double toe taps.* While sitting with the feet flat on the floor, lift the toes off the floor, and then lift the balls of the feet off the floor. Lower in two steps also: First place the balls of the feet on the floor, keeping the toes lifted. Then lower the toes. Do 8 to 12 reps, 1 to 3 sets. Do this daily.
- *Towel scrunch.* Sitting in a chair, spread a hand towel lengthwise on the floor. Starting with the end closest to the foot, use the toes to slowly scrunch the towel, like an accordion. Do twice with each foot.

woven mesh) are usually warmer, and there are shoes with zip-over covers to protect against snow and cold. Be aware that some of these may be heavier or less flexible, affecting gait and performance. If clients notice that this change results in pain or discomfort, they could return to their warmer-weather shoes and always have a pair of dry socks and shoes ready to change into after the walking workout. Many people find that simply changing to warmer socks such as those made out of merino wool is sufficient. If your client stores their shoes in an unheated room or garage, they will stiffen in the cold. Suggest that they find a place to store them indoors during the winter season or bring them inside for at least half an hour before walking.

Lower Body

The options for lower-body apparel are staggering. For warmer weather, there are shorts, cropped pants, and skorts (skirts with shorts sewn underneath). Mostly, choice comes down to personal preference and comfort. If chafing between the thighs is a problem, wearing a skin-tight leg covering like bike shorts (minus the padded butt) that extends to above the knee can help to avoid this irritation. For those who don't like wearing such revealing, form-fitting clothing, regular shorts can be layered over bike shorts.

While some people may wear skin-hugging pants or tights to show off a fit body, experienced walkers have learned that it's more about performance and comfort. Baggy pants, especially those with elastic at the ankles, get hot. The air trapped between the material and the leg has no way to escape, and heat builds. That may be a good thing in winter, but if they are made from material that has any cotton content, the cotton will absorb sweat and become heavy or ungainly and may cause chafing.

Pants that fit more closely to the skin and are made of synthetic material that wicks sweat away from the legs prevent these problems. They also keep the body cooler in warm weather by enhancing the evaporation of sweat—the body's natural air-conditioning. In cold weather, the synthetic material will wick the sweat away from the body so that legs stay drier and warmer.

The fit of tights, especially in the lower leg, is helpful when increasing speed and dealing with bad weather. As walkers get faster, their feet land closer to the midline of the body, compared to typical walking, where they are more parallel to each other. Loose-fitting pants at the ankle can get in the way of that technique, while tights do not. Also, loose pants that fall lower than the heel soak up water and slush when it rains or snows, making walking extremely awkward and uncomfortable. Just like with socks, compression tights are available, but there is little proof that they improve performance during walking, making their high cost hardly justifiable.

As a coach, you can encourage people to try pants or tights that offer greater performance while respecting that each individual will make their own decision based on many factors, including physical and psychological comfort as well as financial budgets.

When the weather gets colder, layering pants creates an air space that might have been too hot in summer but works perfectly as temperatures drop. Windproof pants can create an extra layer of air that adds warmth.

Upper Body

Just like for the lower body, it is possible to fill an entire house with the options for shirts (tank tops, short-sleeve, long-sleeve), pullovers (hooded, zippered), and jackets. Many of these variations are simply a matter of personal preference. Here we discuss the performance and safety concerns.

Sports Bras

While a regular bra may be fine for many women since walking doesn't cause a lot of bouncing, those who experience breast pain during exercise (more than half of women do) should consider a sports bra. The right one can eliminate pain. When British researchers tested 70 women ranging in cup sizes from A to F, they found that encapsulation-style bras, which have separate molded cups, reduced pain the most [3]. This is believed to help because these bras stopped breast motion in all directions, not just up and down. Women needing sizes larger than a D cup should also look for wide straps that offer more back support. Sports bras are usually made with wicking fabric to alleviate any chafing.

Shirts

The principles of what to look for in pants also apply to shirts. A close-fitting shirt made of synthetic wick-away fabric will carry sweat away from the body to encourage cooling in warmer weather and warming in cold weather. As temperatures fall, shirts can be layered to create the air spaces that will increase heat.

For those concerned about sun exposure, clothing can contain SPF (sun protection factor), just like sunscreens. Specialty fabrics have been designed to block the burning ultraviolet (UV) rays of the sun that get through very small holes in the weave of typical fabrics. Purchase clothes that offer a minimum SPF of 30. This allows only 1/30th of the sun's harmful rays to reach the skin. If these shirts seem a little pricey, consider clothing with vibrant colors because they tend to block out more of the sun's rays than lighter color fabrics. Stay away from black and red, because they absorb UVA and UVB rays. Also, washing garments before wearing can shrink the size of the spaces between cloth fibers, letting less sun through to the skin.

Jackets

As the weather cools, layering shirts may not offer sufficient warmth, and people will have to consider wearing jackets. Any jacket will do, but a closer-fitting jacket will allow the arms to move more easily at the shoulder joints. Also, many form-fitting jackets are made from synthetic wick-away materials that will help draw sweat away from the body to keep walkers drier and warmer. On the very coldest days, there may be frost on the outside of these jackets because the sweat that was drawn out has frozen.

One of the challenges of cold-weather walking is feeling warm enough as the walk begins and then managing the heat build-up when the walk becomes vigorous. This has led to features such as hoods, built-in neck warmers, and longer sleeves to cover hands. Once the body warms up, hoods and neck warmers can be pulled off, and hand covers can be folded back. Many jackets also include venting zippers—typically found under the arms—that clients can open as they warm up and close as they cool down at the end of walk. If you live in an area with a lot of precipitation, a waterproof jacket may be a good investment.

Head and Neck

While the myth that we lose most heat through our heads has been busted, there are other valid reasons for covering this area.

Hats

A hat could conceivably be worn all year. A peaked baseball-style cap in warmer weather protects the eyes from sun and rain. This has the effect of improving posture because people wearing peaked caps do not have to bend their heads down to protect the eyes from sun or rain. A wet hat can offer refreshment in hot temperatures. Hats made of wick-away synthetic fabric that offer the same cooling and warming benefits as shirts and pants made out of similar material can be purchased. While heat lost through the head isn't as big of a concern as it was once thought to be, most people will be more comfortable wearing a warm hat during cold weather, especially to help keep their ears warm. As temperatures drop, hats can protect the ears from frostbite.

Alternatives to hats include headbands and visors. Headbands can protect the ears from cold and frostbite. Also, headbands can provide protection from rain for people wearing hearing aids or who have cochlear implants. Visors are a good alternative in the summer for people who find hats too hot but would like eye protection from the sun's rays.

Neck-Warmers

We have noticed that walkers with exposed necks in cold weather tend to have poor posture, hunching their shoulders and pulling their heads forward in an effort to stay warm. A balaclava or neck-warmer (also known as a buff) is essential in cold weather. A neck-warmer is a material tube that is worn around the neck but can be pulled up over the chin and nose to warm the face. A balaclava covers the head and face, leaving just the eyes, nose, and mouth clear. Or, a scarf could be used. When walking in dry, cold air, breathe into the neck-warmer, balaclava, or scarf to allow moist, exhaled air to be breathed back in. This is particularly helpful for people with asthma or heart disease. This warm air will also help keep the nose and cheeks warm—usually the first part of the face that might be affected by frostbite.

The Race Case to Support Walking Divisions

Case Study

The Delaware & Lehigh National Heritage Corridor (D&L) is a multifaceted organization that works to conserve cultural and natural resources along a 165-mile, multiuse trail that runs from the mountains of northeast Pennsylvania down toward Philadelphia. One of its major fundraisers was a marathon and half marathon on the D&L trail. In 2014, the organization dropped the marathon portion and added a walking division to the half marathon. They hired Michele to help make their event walker-friendly.

After creating and running *Prevention* magazine's marathon walking program for five years, participating in races across the country, and talking to hundreds of walkers about their race experiences, Michele had clear ideas for how to create a five-star, walker-friendly half marathon. The leadership at the D&L was completely onboard. If they were going to have a walking division, they wanted to do it right. They completely understood the need to treat walkers and runners as equals. Both are paying the same amount of money to participate and should have a similar experience. Even if a participant is the last one to arrive at a hydration station, they will find water and sports drinks. And, even the last person across the finish line will have hot food and beverages.

The time limit for the D&L Heritage Half Marathon is 4.5 hours, making doing a half marathon possible for both fast and slow walkers. And just like runners, walkers have the chance to win age-group awards. This is quite rare even in races that are supportive of walkers because it is challenging to ensure that people are walking the entire course. In addition to reminding people signing up for the walking division that they must walk every step of the course (no running), each walker wears a bib on the back to easily identify the participants of the walking division. There are pace groups for walkers to help them reach the finish line in a specific amount of time. Also, a walk/run category was created to emphasize the fact that completing a race by alternating running intervals with walking intervals is entirely different than walking the entire race. Anyone registering in the walk/run category receives a runner's bib to distinguish them on the course from walk-only competitors and to ensure they don't take an award from someone registered in the walk-only division.

A driving force behind the change was to increase participation in the event because so many people prefer walking over running. The addition of the walking division has added about 200 participants to an event with a 1,000-person cap and attracted walkers from across the country.

Go to https://race.delawareandlehigh.org for more information.

Lightweight neck-warmers can also be used in the summer when swarms of bugs get thick. It can be pulled up over the nose and mouth so that no bugs are inhaled!

Staying Safe

Personal comfort is a great starting point to ensure that people will enjoy walking and return to class, but safety must always be your priority. Here are tips to ensure that you've thought of everything.

Hydration

At any time of the year, it's a good idea to carry water. For short walks in temperate weather, being hydrated before a walk may be sufficient. For walks that are longer than 60 minutes, especially in the dry conditions that usually accompany extreme cold or in conditions of extreme heat, it is a good idea to encourage people to bring water on walks. While carrying a water bottle in one hand is an option, over even a short amount of time, this asymmetry in the body may lead to muscle imbalance and injury. Similarly, we don't recommend handheld bottle holders because we believe they encourage a lopsided arm gait which may lead to imbalance, discomfort, and injury. Instead, carry a water bottle in a waist pack holder, available at most sporting goods stores. This allows the water bottle to sit comfortably at the front or back of the body, leaving the hands and arms free to swing. As far as water bottles themselves go, there are a range of options. If buying plastic, look for varieties that do not contain BPA. Stainless-steel, insulated versions are helpful in areas that experience either extreme heat or cold. In the heat, put ice in the bottle, and in the cold, pour in hot water.

Visibility

While a walking class provides safety in numbers, if walking after dark or during the early morning or late-evening dusk, darkness presents hazards. People driving cars often complain that they do not see people out walking during these times. Encourage everyone to make themselves visible. Studies have shown that the sooner a driver can see people and the more they are recognizable as human, the safer they will be [4].

Two options for being seen are reflective clothing and lights. With reflective clothing, the headlights of cars are reflected back at drivers, making a walker visible to them. Hats, shirts, jackets, pants, shoes, socks, gloves, and vests are available with embedded reflective material. Or apply reflective tape to clothing. It is important to recognize that the reflective material works only when a light is shining on it. Reflective clothing will not make a walker more visible if a car does not have its headlights on or the headlights are not striking the reflective material.

A second option is to wear lights. There are many lighting options: steady or flashing and in colors such as red, white, or amber. Wear white or amber lights in front of the body, and red or amber lights at the back of the body. This mimics the standard light colors for vehicles. Many lights are now made with rechargeable batteries so that there is less chance that it will burn out during a walk if it is charged after every walk. If using lights with nonrechargeable batteries, be sure to have a good supply of replacement batteries on hand.

We recommend wearing a combination of reflective gear and lights because lights can be seen from a farther distance, and reflective gear can be strategically placed so drivers more easily recognize you as a person rather than as a road marker or another vehicle. The more reflective material on the body to create the shape of a person, the more quickly you will be visible and recognizable to drivers. By placing lights or reflective material on hands, arms, legs, and feet, drivers will see movement, which has been shown in studies to speed recognition.

Even in daylight hours, whether walking in urban, suburban, or rural environments, it is a good idea to wear bright clothing. There is no

Signs of Heat Stroke

The definition of heat stroke is abnormally high body temperature. It should be treated as a medical emergency and can be fatal if not treated properly. Exertional heat stroke can happen quickly, so as a coach, you should be familiar with the following symptoms.

- Fainting
- Headache
- Dizziness
- Cessation of sweating
- Red, hot, dry skin
- Severe fatigue
- Muscle cramps or muscle weakness
- Nausea and vomiting
- Rapid heart rate
- Rapid, shallow breathing
- Confusion
- Unconsciousness

If someone experiences any of these symptoms, move them to a cooler, shady, or air-conditioned place. Call for medical assistance immediately. If possible while waiting for medical assistance, offer something cool to drink, apply ice packs to armpits, groin, neck, and back, or immerse in a cool shower or bath.

significant research on the colors best worn by runners, walkers, and cyclists, but the American National Standard for High-Visibility Safety Apparel and Headwear (ANSI/ISEA 107-2010) recommends the following colors for workers needing safety apparel: fluorescent yellow-green, fluorescent orange-red, and fluorescent red. Fluorescent yellow-green is considered the best choice for daylight and all-round option, while fluorescent orange-red and red are more visible at dusk.

On rural roads, drivers do not expect to see walkers along the side of the road. Bright clothing, or simply a bright safety vest, announce to drivers that you are sharing the road with them. The same is true for suburban areas that do not have sidewalks. Even when walking on sidewalks, bright clothing (and lights at night) help bring awareness to drivers who are pulling cars out of driveways. Neon pink is used often at sea for high visibility and may be a good option for walkers.

Outside Year-Round

While some are lucky to live in temperate climates and experience only small fluctuations in temperature and precipitation, most of us experience cold and heat, rainstorms, possibly hail, snow, thunder, and lightning. On the upside, amazing changes in beauty accompany seasonal change: the bright light of snow in winter; the smell of the thawed earth and new buds in spring; blue skies and flowers in summer; and the burnished reds, oranges, and yellows of leaves in the autumn. We have already reviewed safety and gear; here we take a quick look at how class logistics may change according to the changing temperature and precipitation of the seasons.

When you experience extremes of either cold or heat, you will need to change class organization as a matter of safety as much as participant comfort. Your warm-up, workout, and cool-down will change.

Safety is always your priority. If it is too dangerous to drive to class, to walk in class because of the risk of falls on ice or frostbite, or to breathe because of poor air quality or bitterly cold air, cancel class. Always give people permission to skip class under any condition that compromises their sense of confidence.

Cold

Many people do not enjoy walking in cold weather: anything below 32 degrees F (0 degrees C), and they head indoors to hibernate. Your job as coach is to offer guidance on how to stay warm and provide inspiration for why walking in cold weather improves mood!

Apparel

The great availability and variety of apparel designed to keep us warm in cold weather is helpful. Ideally, winter clothing is made from material that pulls sweat away from the body so that the skin stays dry. The dryness of skin helps maintain warmth. Layering the body, head, hands, and even feet with this technical fabric moves dampness away to the outmost layer and provides air pockets to hold heat close to the body. If people drive to class, encourage them to put dry clothes and boots in the car so they can change into them after the workout.

Frostbite

If temperatures drop below freezing, exposed skin is subject to frostbite. Nonwater-based skin creams such as petroleum jelly, shea butter, or beeswax should be put on exposed skin to protect from frostbite. Eyes should be protected, too. Glasses or ski goggles can be used. Get participants to buddy up and check each other for signs of frostbite—skin will first begin to hurt and turn red, then lose color, appearing white to the observer. When skin has lost color, there will be a loss of feeling. This is why the buddy system is vital to checking for white spots on the skin. If there is any loss of color or white spots, the skin must be covered immediately, and the person should get somewhere warm as soon as possible. Frostbite will permanently damage skin. A severe case to the nose, fingers, and toes may lead to amputation. We love walking during the winter, but the risks associated with frostbite must be taken seriously.

Shoe Ice Grippers

Snow build-up means that walking can get easier if the snow is compacted. Still, walkers can be at risk of slipping and falling. Ice grippers come in a variety of designs, but all can be placed over regular shoes and feature some form of spikes, chain, or metal binding that cover the soles of shoes to dig into soft ice or packed snow. This creates traction. Some shoes contain small spikes for this purpose. They stop people from slipping and falling and even help people maintain speed so that they stay warm and enjoy a good workout.

Hard ice or black ice present a challenge even for ice grippers. A flash freeze makes walking particularly dangerous, and ice grippers do not protect from slipping. The spikes need something to grip, and black ice is too hard for the spikes to sink into. Be on the lookout for patches of black ice and avoid them.

Ice grippers are extremely dangerous indoors, especially on floor surfaces like tile or granite. Always put them on outside; never wear them indoors. You may want to have a few on hand to offer people, because they usually fit over a range of shoe sizes. Lee keeps several in her car and offers them to walkers. She has found that people love how the grippers provide gait and stability confidence, allowing them to enjoy some of the most beautiful winter wonderland walking days.

If you live in an area with a lot of snow or ice, encourage people to bring their own. They can be easily stored in a pocket and put on as needed.

Class Accommodation

In cold weather, encourage all participants to maintain a pace that keeps them warm. When faster people slow down to chat with slower people, they risk having their extremities freeze. Remind them to go as fast as necessary to stay warm; if they get too far ahead, just have them loop back to the main group. Keep the dynamic warm-up sufficiently vigorous to maintain heat in the body. Keep the class moving at all times and possibly shorten the cool-down as body temperatures will drop drastically and quickly when sweating and moving less vigorously. Consider keeping all cool-down stretches dynamic and perhaps shortening class time. If you are fortunate to have an indoor area available, move inside for the cool-down.

Heat

While it sounds inviting, hot weather brings a host of dangers that sometimes cannot be addressed by simply removing layers.

Hydration

As mentioned earlier, staying hydrated at all times is a good idea, but as the temperature rises over 70 degrees F (21 degrees C), hydration is essential. Tell people to arrive to class hydrated and carry extra water, possibly even drinks containing electrolytes. As a coach, it is your responsibility to know where to find drinking fountains or places to refill water bottles along your walking route.

Core Temperature

Even if the body is well hydrated, it can get simply too hot. When core temperature rises above its homeostatic preference of 98.6 degrees F (37 degrees C), the body is experiencing heat stroke. Know the indications of heat stroke (see the Signs of Heat Stroke section earlier in this chapter), and immediately get the person to a cool place and taking in cool liquids.

Sun Protection

On cloudless days in the heat (and sometimes even when it is cool), check the UV index and suggest that people put on sun protection cream or spray before coming to class.

Bugs

As the warm weather arrives, so do bugs and the risk for bug bites that might make people sick. Encourage people to wear bug spray or protective clothing, especially if you are walking in wooded or grassy areas. Everyone should also check themselves for ticks after walking in these types of areas.

Class Accommodation

In hot weather, it will not be necessary to warm up the body. Instead, it will be your job to ease people into movement in a way that helps them acclimatize to the heat. If shade provides relief, look for shaded places where drills can be held. If humidity is high, shade provides little or no respite. Respect that. Whether humidity is high or low, in extreme heat, speed intervals should be spaced by longer recovery periods as hearts will already be stressed by the heat. Verbally cue people to listen to their bodies. If they need to skip intervals, that is a good alternative. If most people are skipping intervals, it's a sign that you are asking too much, and you should consider shortening the class length or do more moderate intervals, such as band exercises while walking (see Walk and Tone drills in chapter 5), stationary strength moves, or balance challenges. Michele has even brought small balls to class on hot days and done tossing drills while walking and standing to challenge eye–hand coordination and balance.

Extreme heat must be taken seriously, especially when combined with high humidity and smog. Under these conditions, the benefits of physical exertion are negated by the stress felt on the body, so always heed local weather advisories in these circumstances. Over 17 years of holding outdoor walking classes, Lee has cancelled only a handful of classes, and these have usually been on "triple alert" days of high heat, humidity, and smog.

Precipitation

Everyone loves a blue-sky day, but precipitation happens. From rainbows to snow-covered trees, precipitation has resulted in some of our most stunning walks over the years. Given that precipitation is often the reason people will stay home from class, it's helpful to have a few ideas that make these walks special. Our best coaching tip for precipitation is to welcome everyone with your biggest smile!

Snow

Snow makes a walk beautiful and memorable. Lee has occasionally been out when there is just a dusting of snow and encouraged people to walk on the pristine snow and then look back to check their footprints in the snow. It's a great visual indicator of foot alignment and stride length. Beautiful, and a helpful teaching tool!

Still, snow can pose safety concerns. Freshly fallen snow can be slippery, especially if it has fallen after a quick freeze, because it may hide black ice. If snow begins to fall during a class, remind people to shorten their stride lengths to keep center of gravity over their feet so that if they do slip, it is easier to recover. A heavy snowfall may require people to change gait to make their way through deep snow. That's OK; it becomes a different kind of workout in which they are doing more quad work as they lift their legs up and out of the snow.

Falling snow can also hinder visibility. Encourage people to wear bright clothing to class and stay off roads. It is possible that drivers may not see you or your class participants, but even if they do, they may brake and slide into people.

During the snowy months in Canada, not all roads are plowed and clear, diminishing the selection for walking routes. Lee often offers hill workout classes during this time of year. Look for a park or road with a hill that is cleared of snow. The effort of walking hill inclines works well to keep people warm in cold weather! There are many variations on hill repeats that can keep people entertained for an entire snowy season (see Hill Intervals section in chapter 5).

Rain

While less problematic than snow, rain can also hinder visibility. Wear bright clothes and be especially vigilant about class participants obeying traffic rules. You'll also want to encourage participants to avoid painted lines on roads since these areas become slippery when wet. Getting wet makes people cold, especially at the end of class, when they are doing less vigorous movement. If you know there is a chance of rain, suggest that participants bring dry clothes to change into after class. If rain is accompanied by lightning and thunder, it is time to end class.

A little rain will not demand a change in class structure. A lot of rain may be different. These are the classes that we typically shorten because soggy feet can lead to blisters. We introduce our most intense intervals: hill repeats and drills that have a competitive nature because we know this type of workout can be as effective as a longer workout. People will leave this shorter rainy class with a sense of accomplishment that is equivalent to a longer fair-weather class.

Whether it's encouraging your walkers to find the gear that works for them or overcoming weather extremes, a creative mindset and persistence are all you need to keep everyone walking. In the next chapter, we'll look at how to set walkers up for success, whether they are simply new to walking or they arrive with medical conditions that are best served with understanding and special consideration.

References

1. Duvall, J. and DeYoung, R. 2013. "Some Strategies for Sustaining a Walking Routine: Insights from Experienced Walkers." *Journal of Physical Activity & Health* 10 (1): 10-18. https://pdfs.semanticscholar.org/0ec5/2f1ac4dc9c5aae0e4af9d39bb8c614dc4c80.pdf.
2. Clinghan, R., Arnold, G.P., Drew, T.S., Cochrane, L.A., and Abboud, R.J. 2008. "Do You Get Value for Money When You Buy an Expensive Pair of Running Shoes?" *British Journal of Sports Medicine* 42 (3): 189-93. www.ncbi.nlm.nih.gov/pubmed/17932096.
3. White, J.L., Scurr, J.C., and Smith, N.A. 2009. "The Effect of Breast Support on Kinetics During Overground Running Performance." *Ergonomics* 52 (4): 492-98. www.ncbi.nlm.nih.gov/pubmed/19401901.
4. Tyrrell, R.A., Wood, J.M., Owens, D.A., Borzendowski, S.W., and Sewall, A.S. 2016. The Conspicuity of Pedestrians at Night: A Review. *Clinical and Experimental Optometry* 99: 425-34. https://onlinelibrary.wiley.com/doi/pdf/10.1111/cxo.12447.

9

Include Everyone

Because walking is accessible to so many people, sedentary to active, you may discover that a wide variety of people have signed up for your program. This could include those who are new to exercise and people who are not new to exercise but are new to vigorous walking. In addition, there may be people with various health conditions for whom walking remains an accessible activity, even interval walk workouts. All these populations will benefit from attending introductory classes. You'll be surprised at how you can accommodate all levels of experience and fitness in the same class.

Introductory classes are an excellent way to introduce both the active and inactive to walking. We always recommend reminding people that learning a new walking technique takes time. Every human has been walking for decades. We have well-established neuropathways from our brains to the muscles used for walking. Everyone in your class will have a unique gait based on anatomy and factors such as work, past injury, whether they are male or female, and so much more. People who have been completely sedentary may notice the greatest benefits in the shortest amount of time. For those who are already fit from other activities, it may take longer to realize new benefits because they first need to master the technique in order to challenge themselves enough to see improvements, especially for cardiorespiratory fitness.

There are special populations for whom walking provides an accessible way to get exercise. We review several possibilities here, but any person coming to class should complete a health questionnaire (see appendix B) so that you are fully aware of any potential challenges. If you are unfamiliar with a particular health risk, ask if they have ever had any specific recommendations from a health professional regarding activity. For example, Lee was once walking with a new client who required regular sips of water because of an autoimmune disease that causes an extremely dry mouth. Lee was unfamiliar with the condition but learned that it required constant hydration. The client was perfectly capable of meeting her needs, but it was a signal for Lee to ask more questions and be alert for signs of discomfort, fatigue, or breathlessness that might warrant a reduction in exertion level.

Pay special attention to complaints about pain. Many of us experience pain at some point, whether it be in a muscle or at a joint, and more often than not, it goes away. Ongoing pain is not normal. (See How Exercise

Tracking Daily Steps

It's become commonplace to hear recommendations to walk 10,000 steps every day so it's possible that your clients are tracking their steps or thinking about it. So what advice should you give them?

Let them know that this is not a magic number. Of course, walking 10,000 steps a day is likely to help them to feel better and be healthier. When sedentary folks increased their daily step count to 10,000, they were 46% less likely to die during a four-year study than those who remained sedentary, according to an Australian study published in the journal *Plus One* [1]. But 10,000 may not be the right number for everyone—and benefits have been seen with even small increases of 2,000 to 3,000 steps a day. So, tracking steps is worth the investment in a pedometer or activity tracker. Dozens of studies have reported that people who track their steps, increase the number that they take by up to 3,500 steps per day [2].

People in professions such as nursing might already reach 10,000 steps most days of the week. If they want to see improvements, they will have to go higher to challenge their bodies and see changes. Others may be getting only 3,000 to 4,000 a day, so 10,000 may seem impossible. To help your walkers find the right personal step goal, encourage them to start by getting a baseline of how many steps they're currently taking. The objective of this exercise is for them to go through their usual daily routine—without trying to walk more than they normally do. If they already walk regularly, it's probably a good idea to do a baseline on both a day when they take a structured walk, and on a day when they don't. They should track at least two weekdays and one weekend day. Once they have their baseline number, encourage them to increase their steps about 1,000 to 2,000 each day for a week. The next week, bump the goal up another 1,000 to 2,000 steps. Continue this until they reach at least 10,000 steps a day. If weight loss is their goal, getting even more steps will speed up results.

Keep in mind that step counts don't account for intensity. Encourage your clients to get a portion of their steps each day in a set amount of time, for example 3,750 steps in 30 minutes to ensure some of the steps are taken at a brisk pace and enhance benefits. (See the Steps to Speed section in chapter 3 to help you calculate recommendations.)

Should Feel in chapter 3.) If you notice someone consistently complaining, suggest that they see a health professional.

While you may need to make accommodations for certain populations, it is our experience that many people do not need to be treated specially and indeed do not want to be singled out. We encourage you to be confident that if a person has expressed interest in walking class, they have a certain level of confidence that they are capable of participating. Trust that walking is going to improve stamina while staying alert to potential risks and organizing the class in such a way that everyone feels included.

Introductory Class

All participants are served well by learning good walking technique. An introductory program or class can do this and also offers an opportunity to review the basics of interval training and the looping technique (see Learn to Loop section in chapter 5). Even very fit participants will get more from their walking after such a class or series of classes. If someone interested in joining your walking program cannot attend an intro session, suggest that they try a regular walking workout class. If they enjoy it, they could keep attending the workout classes and may pick up the basics of technique through doing the drills. Suggest they attend an intro class at some point to get a comprehensive overview of walking technique.

Walking Technique

The four progressions of good walking technique outlined in chapter 4 should be covered in any introductory session. There are many ways to manage this introductory session depending on your participants, the season, your location, and more. For example, you could offer a two-hour workshop, although that is a short time to cover all four progressions. A four- or eight-week introductory session that consists of 45- or 60-minute classes works well, allowing you to introduce one progression each week and give people time to practice that progression after class and before the next class. This might be ideal in a work environment for classes held during a lunch hour.

Benchmark Walk

A benchmark walk involves timing people over a set distance or setting a time for people to walk a distance as a way for them to see their progress. We suggest including a benchmark walk as part of an intro class because it offers a concrete and rewarding way for participants to see how walking speed increases just by introducing one or more of the technique progressions. Doing this once at the beginning of an intro class or program after the warm-up and a second time at the end of class or the program before the cool-down provides a gratifying sense of success and boost in confidence. In all our years coaching hundreds of clients, we've had only one time where someone was slower—and she had another success that was more meaningful to her. For the story, see chapter 4.

We recommend doing the benchmark drill in your introductory class in a way that avoids a single starting line. This may be stressful for people who are new to exercise because it feels too competitive. Instead, have everyone choose a different place to stand as a starting point. They should identify this point by a marker, perhaps leaving a twig by the side of their position. Or, bring a box of colorful chalk to class and have everyone draw a start mark on the pavement. If you live in an area where chalk would not be washed away by rain, you may want to consider simply placing stones or other natural markers at the start and finish instead of using chalk. From this starting point, have them walk as fast as they can for anywhere from 30 to 45 seconds, putting an item on the ground to mark their finish point or using their chalk to do so. After you have taught them some or all the walking progressions, have them repeat the drill. They will usually walk farther in the same amount of time. It is an encouraging method to have people experience success in their first class while also learning the value of good walking technique.

Benchmark walks can also be used over a session of classes or at regularly scheduled times during the course of a year. Tracking these extended periods is a great way to show participants the value of regularly attending walking workout classes. It can be motivating when they might be discouraged. For example, in a class environment, you may have the same participants each week, so everyone improves over an eight-week session. Both faster and slower walkers get faster, but the slower walkers may not realize it because they are still behind the faster walkers. Recorded benchmark times reveal how much faster they are in objective terms, with slower walkers often seeing greater improvements. If you plan to track results over the course of an entire session of classes or every six months, you'll want to record time rather than distance. Use an established route, such as a track, looped path in a park, or a specific segment of a road so that you can return to the same spot in the future. We suggest a timed mile as a good distance for this.

Speed Intervals

Even in an introductory class, it can be fun and helpful to invite the participants to do speed intervals. Picking up the pace helps walkers get a sense of how to integrate the ideas about technique into fast walking. It also shows them how good form and technique improve speed. And, finally, doing these speed bursts in an introductory class ensures that participants leave having increased their heart rates—giving them a taste of the energy kick of vigorous walking!

Here is an example of an interval workout for a first class that helps to reinforce good walking techniques. At the beginning of each interval, have participants focus on a specific walking technique while they walk as fast as possible (see chapter 4, Progressions 2 and 3 for more technique descriptions). This series of four intervals could be repeated two or three times, depending on the reception by the participants. If they seem to be enjoying it, go for three sets!

- 30-seconds: heel strike (toe up) and straight leg landing
- 30-seconds: butt squeeze action
- 30-seconds: shortened stride and quickened leg turnover (faster leg cadence)
- 30-seconds: elbow punch back

If you are teaching a six- to eight-week session of introductory classes in which you are introducing only one or two aspects of technique each week, you could repeat intervals focusing on the same technique, such as bending your arms, each interval. Or you could mix some technique suggestions into some of the shorter go-recover drills offered in chapter 5.

Seniors

Technically, anyone over age 65 is considered a senior, even though we have found that number to be deceiving. Age is a state of mind, and many walkers over 65 are inspirational to those who are younger. When people join Lee's program, she does not ask their ages, and sometimes, upon learning it, she has been surprised to have thought the person is 10 or 15 years younger than they are.

Still, common physical changes happen to even healthy seniors, all of which should be covered in your health questionnaire.

- High blood pressure: Many people over 50, especially if they are carrying even modest extra weight, have high blood pressure for which they are taking medication, or they may have been referred to an exercise program by their family doctor. There are over 450 different medications for blood pressure that fall in a range of categories, including diuretics, beta blockers, ACE inhibitors, angiotensin II receptor blockers, calcium channel blockers, and much more. Several of these can artificially lower heart rate readings. It is probably easiest to simply ask if they are taking medication to control blood pressure, and if so, ask if their doctor has suggested exercising to a specific heart rate or according to RPE. Watch for excessive redness of the face, sweating, and severe shortness of breath that might indicate cardiorespiratory distress.

- Glaucoma: Open-angle glaucoma is characterized by damage to the optic nerve, most often caused by high intraocular pressure, and it is common in people over 65. Daily drops or surgery may be prescribed, but it does not cure the damage, and doctors will recommend that patients keep their heads over their hearts to prevent the increased pressure that happens when the head is lower than the heart. This is something to keep in mind if you include any strength or stretch moves in class. Keep heads higher than hearts. Also, holding the breath during strength exercises may increase intraocular pressure, just as it may increase blood pressure in general. Repeated reminders to breathe are helpful, especially if you incorporate strength moves in a walking class.

- Loss of bone density: This is common as people age, particularly for small people who carry little to no excess weight. Weight bearing exercise (especially fast interval walking) has the potential to strengthen bone density, but it is good to keep in mind that people with low bone density may be at greater risk for a fracture after a seemingly innocuous stumble and even stress fractures from overuse.

Chronic Leg and Foot Issues

Injured knees, backs, and feet are common reasons that people who were previously active in other sports, such as running, join walking programs. In chapter 4, we discussed how good walking form can help to strengthen the muscles that support the low back and knees. Encourage clients who may have low-back or knee issues to maintain their best walking form according to the progressions laid out. It can be tempting during interval drills (especially self-compete drills) to work so hard that form is compromised, and the risk of injury goes up. If participants face recurring issues with any joints, including those at the back, hips, knees, or feet, it is always a good idea to suggest they visit a health specialist. Pain or discomfort is not normal, and there are usually ways to address it so people can continue walking comfortably.

Foot injuries can pose a special challenge as it is sometimes difficult to allow feet the rest they need to heal. Two typical issues that we come across frequently in our class participants include bunions and plantar fasciitis.

Bunions

A bunion is a bony bump at the base of the toe and from where the toe tends to shift position to angle toward the other toes. Bunions can be extremely painful for people when doing any activity that requires weight on the bunion. Also, it can be difficult to find shoes that are comfortable.

In his book, *The Science of Yoga: The Risks and the Rewards*, William J. Broad describes the work of New York City orthopedic surgeon, Loren Fishman, who recommends that people with bunions or a tendency to develop bunions do the following exercise daily: Pull the big toe away from the second toe and then let it return to its resting position. Repeat pulling the big toe to the side and letting it return to its resting position for 20 to 30 seconds each day. This is worth trying if it means avoiding surgery!

Surgery to cure bunions is extremely painful and requires at least four to six weeks of recovery, although we have had many people return to walking programs pain-free after the surgery, even walking marathons.

Plantar Fasciitis

Plantar fasciitis is inflammation-causing pain in the connective tissue that supports the bottom of the foot, and it is characterized by pain in the sole of the foot at the heel, particularly upon placing the foot on the ground first thing in the morning. It is typically thought that plantar fasciitis is caused by overuse, and a common recommendation is to simply stay off the feet for them to heal—not always a feasible solution! Other tips include putting on a supportive shoe before the heel hits the ground in the morning and leaving it on until going to bed at night, rolling the foot on a frozen water bottle, and stretching the gastrocnemius and the soleus muscles (see lower body exercises in chapter 6). Another healing option is to sit with the affected foot resting on the opposite thigh. Pull the toes of that foot toward the shin until a stretch is felt along the bottom of the foot. Practice self-massage using the thumb or fingers of the opposite hand along the taut band of tissue that can be felt at the sole of the foot.

Plantar fasciitis usually heals with conservative treatment such as that described above, but it commonly takes from six months to a year, which can be frustrating. It is definitely worth seeing a health professional such as a podiatrist for accurate diagnosis and treatment. One alternative for activity is walking in pools to keep the walking muscles strong but eliminate weight bearing on the heel.

Pregnancy and Postnatal

Health professionals encourage walking through pregnancy and in the months immediately following. When pregnant, women experience an increase in blood volume that makes them fatigue easily. Also, joints become less stable and at risk for strains or sprains. Most of these clients will be able to self-monitor for comfort and health. Your role as coach should be to respect their limitations while encouraging them to stay active.

Diabetes

It is common to have people in class with blood sugar challenges ranging from manageable hypoglycemia to the volatile swings in blood sugar of diabetes. The body's response to regular exercise is improved insulin sensitivity, so doctors often recommend walking to people with any insulin insensitivity. Some people manage diabetes with diet and exercise, and others take regular insulin injections or have pumps with continuous glucose monitor patches. It has been our experience that people with severe diabetes come to class well prepared with sugar tablets or juice in case they experience a serious sugar low. Still, it may be a good idea to have something like this on hand. Always pay close attention for any signs that a person is experiencing a sugar low, including shakiness, rapid heart rate, excessive perspiration, and anxiety. They might say that they are dizzy, or they may be walking or speaking erratically. Simply slowing down may help, or they may need to sit down and take in some sugar.

Neurological, Neuromuscular, or Autoimmune Diseases

Many illnesses are rooted in neurological or neuromuscular degeneration or autoimmune dysfunction. Exercise can improve quality of life, even if it does not play a specific role in healing. Again, let your clients take the lead in their ability to do drills. If you are leading interval intensity drills, it might be helpful for them to skip a few. People with many of these illnesses such as multiple sclerosis, amyotrophic lateral sclerosis (ALS), Parkinson's disease, rheumatoid arthritis, or early stages of dementia have better days and worse days. Monitor their situations. Challenge them on a good day, and encourage them to reduce effort on other days.

Osteoarthritis

A high percentage of participants over age 40 will have some form of arthritis in the knees, hips, or feet. For some it will be symptomatic, and they will experience pain. A common recommendation is to rate this pain on a scale of 1 to 10. Ask them if they have been given specific instructions from the doctor pertaining to restrictions or recommendations for physical activity. We have found that teaching good walking form and reinforcing it through drills and cueing works well to help people manage the challenge of osteoarthritis, building muscle stability around the joints that protect them from strain and pain. Another alternative, based on research, may be slow uphill walking (see the Overweight and Obesity section later in this chapter). Encourage any clients with osteoarthritis to talk to their doctors about managing pain during exercise. One of Michele's clients walked through knee pain with her doctor's guidance and was able to avoid knee surgery.

Overweight and Obesity

With more than 70 percent of US adults either overweight or obese, some of them are likely to be your clients, and you need to be ready to offer modifications when necessary. Carrying excess weight affects walking in a number of ways, including creating greater instability that then causes compensatory muscles to work harder, possibly leading to more discomfort or even injury. This, along with having to move more body weight, can result in slower speeds and quicker fatigue. It can also result in more joint issues. If overweight or obese clients—or any clients—are having knee issues when they try to walk faster, an alternative workout may be uphill walking. When Colorado State University researchers tested 12 obese individuals, they found that they got just as good of a workout walking slowly uphill as they did walking faster on level ground. They also found that the load on their knees was lower when walking uphill. Forces on the knee were reduced up to 26 percent when they walked on a 6 degree incline at 1.7 miles per hour (35 min per mile) compared to walking 3.4 miles per hour (18 min per mile) on level ground [3]. This doesn't help if they're walking outdoors since they usually have to return downhill, which can be tough on knees. But it makes a case for training these clients on a treadmill, where they can avoid the downhill. Or encourage them to do this on days when they aren't with you. Depending upon the degree of obesity and mobility issues, these clients may need more emotional support and encouragement. Remind them that doing even a little bit is a big accomplishment. The rewards of the effort can be amazing. We have had overweight and obese clients go on to walk in full and half marathons. One of them has completed over 80 half marathons in just six years while still being obese, so remember that every client is capable of exceeding expectations—especially with your guidance.

Asthma

People who experience asthma may present one of your greatest challenges. Pollution, pollen, high heat, and extreme cold can all trigger asthma attacks, and pushing through symptoms is not appropriate. While many people with asthma are well versed in how to manage it, often the only solution during times of high pollution, pollen, and heat is to stay indoors and walk on a treadmill. The cold of outdoor winter can sometimes be helped by wearing a neck-warmer. By pulling it up over the nose and mouth, participants can breathe in warm moist air from their own exhalations. If someone does experience an asthma attack in class, remember that stress exacerbates the response. Remain calm, ask them if they have medication, and look for signs of extreme distress, such as a blue tinge to skin, lips, or fingernails. Be prepared to call for emergency help.

Even without asthma, the respiratory system can be severely stressed under conditions of high heat, high humidity, and high pollution. We recommend cancelling classes if all three conditions exist. Monitor the effect of any of the three on participants and change class appropriately by reducing the number of intervals, offering longer RPs to WPs, introducing extra stretching, moving to a shaded area, or simply cutting class short.

Visual or Hearing Impairment

You might be surprised at what visually impaired individuals can do (see the case study in this chapter). For people who have some degree of vision impairment, wearing brightly colored clothes as a coach can be helpful. You can be easily seen and followed. Lee has worked with visually impaired individuals with success, although typically in locations that are relatively free from traffic or obstacle concerns, such as wide, paved pedestrian paths. For people who have seriously limited vision or no vision at all, we recommend finding a volunteer guide. Both the guide and the visually impaired walker wear a belt of some sort to which an elastic resistance band can be attached. They can then walk beside each other with their arms and hands free because the band is keeping them connected with slight tension. Still, cuing a visually impaired walker as a guide is a skill that needs development. It involves not just visual acuity but good timing in terms of vocalizing potential hazards. As a coach, you may want to volunteer to be a guide to understand the nuances involved.

A participant with hearing loss is at risk of stepping into traffic and often cannot hear verbal instructions. Try to stay within their hearing range or in front of them so that they can receive visual cues. It is particularly important that walkers with hearing impairment follow conventional rules of the road and pathways. They should walk facing traffic on roads with no sidewalks and walk to the right on shared cycling/pedestrian paths because they are unable to hear cars honking or cyclists ringing bells.

Visually Impaired Walker Gains Self-Confidence From Power Walking

Case Study

At age 73, Arlene Mawson was a true inspiration as she power walked across the finish line of the 2018 Toronto Sporting Life 10K in 1 hour and 28 minutes (about a 14-minute-per-mile pace), finishing in the top half of her age category along with runners. Her accomplishment became even more astonishing when you saw *Blind Walker* on her racing bib. She was tethered to a guide.

Arlene started walking with a personal trainer as her guide in 2006 while in Florida for the winter. At the time, she could make out contrasting surfaces on the ground and light versus shadow around her. Upon returning home to Toronto that spring, Arlene entered the walking division of a popular 10K race and, with a guide, finished 28th out of 226 competitors. She was hooked!

Arlene joined Lee's power walking class, and she recruited friends to become her guides. (Lee does not charge a fee for guides in classes, but they do pay race entry fees.) While walking together, both Arlene and her guide wear waist packs and loop an elastic resistance band to each other's waist packs. This allows both walker and guide to swing their arms freely while still sensing their proximity to each other through the tension in the band. When needed, the guide will reach for Arlene's arm to navigate her away from obstacles. Over the years, her vision has become more impaired due to retinitis pigmentosa, but Arlene has total confidence in her guides and claims that she is more relaxed than they are!

Two of her long-term and consistent guides, Libby McHardy-Hall and Elaine Selke, had no experience guiding before walking with Arlene. One of the trickiest aspects to learning to guide a visually impaired walker is expanding the perception of personal space to include the space of the person being guided. Over the years, Libby and Elaine have developed specific cuing language to quickly alert Arlene to obstacles in her path.

With her guides, Arlene has become a veteran of many races, including half and full marathons. "Power walking has changed my life," she says. "I have gained self-confidence from doing races, and I enjoy the social aspect." Her guides agree, and they add that people often point to them as sources of inspiration.

Cancer (During and After Treatment)

Physical activity is helpful through and beyond cancer treatment. Studies show that it lowers symptoms from treatment, such as fatigue and nausea, and improves five-year survival rates. Any walking class participant going through treatment should determine what intensity and duration works for them, keeping in mind that this may change day-by-day and during different phases of treatment. The most common issue we have experienced over the years is that women who have had mastectomies for breast cancer treatment may experience lymphedema in the arm of that side, especially if lymph nodes have been removed. It can be painful to bend the arm for walking. Many will wear compression bandages to help with this.

Cardiac Concerns

As with many other many health situations, exercise is often prescribed for people with heart disease or who are recovering from a cardiac event. This is because exercise is the best medicine. Take your cues from the participant, and ask them if their doctor has given them any specific instructions pertaining to restrictions or recommendations for physical activity. Most of them will have already participated in cardiac rehabilitation with specialists. Offering longer warm-ups and cool-downs are a good idea. Stopping abruptly may lead to dizziness or lightheadedness. Vigorous SS and HIIT (with longer RPs to WPs) is appropriate. Check in after a series of intensity intervals to confirm that a two-minute recovery finds them speaking easily. People with cardiac issues also need to be more cautious during weather extremes because these types of conditions stress the heart more than exercising during milder weather.

There is always a way to get walking. We have given solutions to common challenges in this chapter. In the next chapter, we'll look at ways to set up and manage your classes so that they work from a variety of coaching perspectives, in a range of locations, and throughout all seasons.

References

1. Ehlen, K.A., Reiser, R.F., and Browning, R.C. 2011. "Energetics and Biomechanics of Inclined Treadmill Walking in Obese Adults." *Medicine & Science in Sports & Exercise* (43) 7: 1251-59. www.ncbi.nlm.nih.gov/pubmed/21200344.
2. Dwyer, T., Pezic, A., Sun, C., Cochrane, J., Venn A., Srikanth, V., Jones, G., Shook, R., Sui, X., Ortaglia, A., Blair, S., and Ponsonby, A.L. 2015. "Objectively Measured Daily Steps and Subsequent Long-Term All-Cause Mortality: The Tasped Prospective Cohort Study." *PLOS One* 10 (12): e0141274. https://journals.plos.org/plosone/article?id=10.1371/journal.pone.0141274.
3. Kanejima, Y., Kitamura, M., and Izawa, K.P. 2018. "Self-Monitoring to Increase Physical Activity in Patients With Cardiovascular Disease: A Systemic Review and Meta-analysis." *Aging Clinical and Experimental Research.* https://link.springer.com/article/10.1007%2Fs40520-018-0960-7#citeas.

PART V

THE BUSINESS OF WALKING

10

Manage Your Classes

If you're reading this book, you likely feel inspired to help people use walking to transform their fitness. In order to go from "inspiration" to "action," let's talk about setting up for success. Your planning needs to support your enthusiasm. Build it properly, and they will come. In this chapter, we'll consider your starting point and review the basic requirements as you launch your walking program.

Determine the Best Approach for Your Goals and Situation

There are a variety of ways to set up a walking program or business to suit your experience, motivation, and audiences. Let's take a moment to consider what the different starting points might be. This will guide you to the most pertinent information in this chapter. Look for the scenario in the following that most closely matches your current situation.

You Have Fitness or Wellness Expertise

Walking programs can be incorporated into your core offerings, or they can be the focus of your programming. Depending upon your current setup, you may not need our suggestions for pricing and website development; however, the information on coaching credentials, scheduling, safety, logistics of walking classes in your location, and promotion will be important as you venture into a new area of programming.

You Have a Solid Client Base

In a corporate, college, or institutional wellness environment, it will be straightforward to introduce a walking program, especially if the environment around your location is walk-friendly. In most cases, programming is offered at no additional charge to employees, faculty, students, or members, so you don't need to set a pricing structure. But you will need an understanding of your audience as well as an appreciation for logistical concerns, such as where and when to walk.

If you own a gym or yoga studio, walking workouts will be an excellent addition to your programming and may be an opportunity to attract individuals who are intimidated by traditional fitness offerings. Much of the information in this chapter will help you introduce it successfully. In addition to the logistical information, you may be interested in the recommendations for pricing and even website organization.

Do you work for or own a wellness, chiropractic, or nutrition business and want to support clients beyond your specialized treatments? A walking program is a perfect way to add a fitness aspect to your services. If your outside environment is suitable for walking, you can do it from your office, no matter how small it is. Promotion can be done through the typical channels you currently use to keep in touch with your clients. If you're hiring a certified coach to lead the program, you may want to charge a fee. You will find the tips on coaching and pricing in this chapter helpful.

You Are Starting or Growing a Business

For group fitness leaders, personal trainers, health coaches, or other fitness and wellness professionals building a business with minimal capital investment, walking offers many options. Walking programs appeal to a wider audience than traditional fitness programming because it's more accessible, giving you a way to tap into the approximately 80 percent of the population who are sedentary or not active enough to meet current guidelines. Because of walking's low cost and low-risk profile, it may be a perfect option if you are interested in booking corporate or health care clients. Your education and training give you a great start on using this book as a resource to create a business based on walking workouts or to include walking workouts as one aspect of your programming. You may want to test the waters by simply offering one class a week in your community. If it is popular, you could expand your course offerings and support your growth with a website, advertising, and marketing, using the suggestions in this chapter.

You Have a Passion for Walking, but No Fitness or Wellness Experience or Credentials

Have you caught the walking bug and would like to see formal walking workouts offered in your community? Do you have friends who enjoy walking together? Could you recruit people through a parent group, book club, local advocacy group, or sports team? If you have no intention of creating a business, the information for pricing and website organization may not be relevant, but the information on coaching as well as the safety and logistics of when and where you walk will be a great starting point to creating a safe and fun local walking program. It's also recommended that you obtain insurance to protect yourself from any liability if any accidents happen (see the Insure Your Business section later in this chapter for more on insurance). The section about coaching requirements will be important information for you to review, along with all the other content in the section.

Whatever your organizational starting point, let's look at the factors that are foundational to creating a successful walking program.

Runner Turned Walking Coach

Case Study

Judy Heller found her way to becoming a walking coach through running. When she repeatedly developed injuries in her feet, knees, and hips, Judy decided that running wasn't going to work for her, and she took up racewalking. To her surprise, she placed in her age group and qualified for big races. "I could achieve in walking what I never could do in running," says Judy, who's competed nationally and internationally. As she became more competitive, friends asked her to coach them. She decided to get her personal training certification to ensure that she provided a high level of coaching. That was more than 25 years ago.

Judy's business, Wonders of Walking, has evolved over the years. In addition to offering walking-specific services, such as classes on technique, instruction on racewalking and Nordic walking (using poles), and training to walk distance events, Judy is also a racewalking judge. For many years, she organized walking events and served as the walking coordinator for the Portland to Coast Walk Relay (part of the Hood to Coast Relay) for nine years. She was the racewalk coordinator for the Portland Marathon, one of the most walker-friendly events in the country, for 18 years. Judy has been a walk coach for the American Diabetes Association's Team Diabetes marathon training program and the Arthritis Foundation's Joints in Motion program.

Judy's business never focused solely on walking; she always incorporated all aspects of fitness, such as stretching and strength training. But over time, as Judy accrued additional training and certifications, she expanded to a total wellness approach, offering lifestyle coaching and nutritional counseling along with her personal training and walking services. No matter what services Judy provides to clients, she always incorporates walking into the programs as her go-to cardio option. "Walking is our default gait and something everyone can do," says Judy, who is still walking and coaching at age 73.

"To really be successful with walking programs, you need to be passionate about walking," Judy says. "You need to look at walking as an athletic endeavor. You have to embrace it. There's an art to walking, just like anything else."

For more information about Judy and Wonders of Walking, go to www.wondersofwalking.com.

Earn Your Coaching Credentials

Educated, knowledgeable, and inspired coaches are the foundation of your success. At present, there are no national standards or credentials for walking coaches. Anyone can call themselves a walking coach. For avid walkers who are keen to start a local walking group and professionals in the fitness industry, there is very little help out there to get started. That is why we wrote this book. Our intention is to offer as much information as possible that will make you the best possible walking coach you can be.

Obviously, as fitness professionals ourselves, we believe in the value of being certified by a national fitness instructor standard with respected organizations for fitness and health, such as American College of Sports Medicine (ACSM), American College of Exercise (ACE), National Strength & Conditioning Association (NSCA), National Academy of Sports Medicine (NASM), Canadian Fitness Professionals (Canfitpro), and National Coaching Certification Program (NCCP, Canada). Consider that most gyms will accept only certifications that are accredited by the National Commission for Certifying Agencies (NCCA).

The knowledge gained through a recognized and accredited certification in terms of exercise physiology and anatomy offers valuable information that can help you develop safe and effective programs, design creative drills, and deal with injury and other challenges. Also, note that many insurance companies will require that you hold current professional certifications with one of these respected organizations in order to be covered by their policies.

However, we also recognize the value of avid walkers or community leaders without formal fitness training. These leaders can create walking programs to motivate the millions of people who are sedentary or not meeting recommended physical activity guidelines to be more active. For an example, check out GirlTrek's story in the chapter 12 case study.

We recommend that, as a minimum, coaches have current certification in cardiopulmonary resuscitation (CPR). There is every reason to sign up for a CPR course. It's a great life skill, and it will make you feel more confident as a leader, giving you basic skills in responding to a health emergency.

Insure Your Business

As safe as walking can be as an activity, if you are organizing or leading walking programs, insurance is necessary. While it is common to develop positive relationships with clients and be lulled into a sense of complacency that they would never sue you, the reality is that they could. If a client believes they were injured from walking, they could file a lawsuit against you. Even if you require walkers to fill out health questionnaires and sign waivers, these documents will not protect you against litigation. If sued successfully, your personal assets may be at risk of loss, depending on your business tax classification. Even if it's not successful, fighting a lawsuit is expensive unless you have insurance. There are a few types of insurance to investigate.

- **Professional liability insurance**, also known as malpractice insurance, protects walking coaches from a client's claim that they were injured as a direct result of coaching advice. Suggesting that a client walk 10 hill repeats twice a week may work well for thousands of clients, but one may experience back pain from a workout and take you to court over it. Moreover, if you plan to hold your walking programs under the auspices of a gym, club, workplace, or other organization, they may demand to see proof of your professional liability insurance. Ask your insurer if they provide a certificate of insurance (COI).

- **General liability insurance** protects you from property damage and personal injury due to accidents that happen while you are leading a walking group, but they are unrelated to your advice. The likelihood of property damage during walking classes is low, especially if programs are held outside. However, personal injury may happen, for example, if someone trips, whether inside or outside.
- **Product liability insurance** may be a good idea if you use any products, such as elastic resistance bands, during walk circuit classes and this is not covered in your general liability insurance. Product liability insurance protects you against any claims arising from injury related to equipment failure.
- **Personal liability insurance** protects against claims from a third party who may be adversely affected by an injury to one of your clients from advice that you gave.
- **Sexual misconduct liability insurance** is a good idea for any person working intimately with others. While you may feel that your own conduct makes this unnecessary, especially in outdoor group settings, it remains an excellent protection in case a client's interpretation of events differs from your own. If you have coaches who lead walking workouts on your behalf, ensure that they are covered, too.
- **Disability insurance** for yourself as a personal trainer or fitness leader dependent on your walking or fitness program for income. This is important when your monthly bills depend on your coaching revenue and you can no longer coach because you are injured.

There are literally hundreds of companies that offer insurance to personal trainers. Check for discounts through such fitness certification organizations as ACE, NASM, ACSM, and NSCA. Some plans offer monthly payment options; however, you may be able to get a price reduction by paying annually. Before making your final purchase on insurance, check for any exclusions. For example, make sure that if you have a substitute coach who does not have a fitness certification, they are covered in event of an accident. Verify that you are covered in all outdoor environments, including on all outdoor roads, trails, sidewalks, intersections, and parking lots—both public and private spaces. If you train virtually, make sure that you are covered. If you teach a yoga pose in walking class, ensure you are covered for that!

Finally, if anything changes in your walking program or business, check back with your insurance provider. This includes any changes to number of classes, number of participants, location, coaches, and equipment used.

Establish Pricing

If you need to make money from your walking program, how you price it may make or break your decision to proceed. If you set up programs for institutions and do not actively recruit individual participants from your local community, it might be better to negotiate a contract based on either an hourly rate or a per-person fee. These may vary, depending on whether you are working with nonprofit or for-profit organizations. Keep in mind that if any of your classes have more than 15 to 20 participants, you may want to work with another coach so that you have a student-to-coach ratio that allows for quality coaching and a safe experience. Keep in mind that your pricing may need to reflect the extra coaching, unless the increased number of participant registrations covers it. Of course, your experience and comfort managing large groups may allow you to lead groups larger than 20 people. And, locations with minimal safety concerns may also make it easier for one coach to manage a larger group. For example, groups of 25 or more may work well at a track.

If you want to recruit participants from the community as you would for typical classes such as yoga and CrossFit, your pricing is a critical competitive component of your plan. If you lead an outdoor program and have no overhead costs of a physical location, it is tempting to underprice your course. Remember that there is value in your education, experience, and motivational skills. Choose a price that reflects this value and know that people will pay for it. If your price is too low as you start your group or business, it will be difficult to bring the price up to align with appropriate reimbursement for your time, experience, and skills. Research the prices of fitness and yoga classes in local gyms and studios. Be sure to check their rates for drop-in classes as well as session pricing and memberships. Consider a pricing structure that is similar or a little lower per class to account for your lack of facility overhead costs. Membership or group pricing is always popular.

How Much to Charge?

Deciding how much to charge for programs or classes can be stressful, especially when it comes to pricing an activity like walking because everyone knows how to do it and can easily do it on their own. Price yourself too high, and people may think it's too expensive. Discount your rates too much, and you may end up feeling resentful and not valued. We've both been there and done that. Through those experiences, we've come up with pricing models that are different, but they work for each of us. If you want to generate revenue from coaching people to walk, we hope our examples will help you set pricing.

Lee has been offering walking workout classes for 17 years and coaching individual clients in person and online. Over the years, she has also had contracts to lead walking workouts at local corporate offices; however, the bulk of her revenue is generated through weekly classes.

Michele has been coaching walking clients for 13 years, but she had been doing so independently for only five years. Her early years of coaching were done online as the fitness director at *Prevention* magazine. Even after she left her corporate position, many of her early coaching jobs were contract positions, in which the company or organization compensated Michele, and participants paid little or no fee for the program.

How Lee Sets Class Pricing

Living in a large metropolitan area, Lee does a casual survey of the pricing at local gyms and yoga studios. Because all her walking classes are held outside, she reduces the average per class fee. This determines a drop-in fee. From there, she reduces the per class fee in a ranked way, depending on the volume and commitment shown by people to register. The next lower level of pricing is the purchase of a six-class pass (which has time restrictions for use), and the per class rate is less than a drop-in rate.

This reduction in rate continues, depending on volume and time commitment to the program. The prices shown in table 10.1 are per class. Classes are either 60 or 90 minutes long, and the price per class is the same for both.

All these options are available for purchase online through her business website. As a courtesy to her ongoing clients, Lee offers a "flash sale" on two-month and four-month all-class passes that is available for just a few days with payment by Interac transfer only.

TABLE 10.1 **Pricing Example***

Drop-in class	6-class pass	8-week session	2-month, 2 classes/week	2-month, 3 classes/week	4-month, 2 classes/week	4-month, 3 classes/week
$16	$14	$13	$11	$10	$10	$9

*Pricing shown in US dollars.

How Michele Sets Pricing

Some drop-in class rates are as low as $5 in Michele's area. This is a perfect example of why it's important to survey your area—so you can set competitive pricing. Since Michele doesn't offer ongoing classes, only 10 to 20 percent of her business focuses on training clients, and she lives in a smaller town, her pricing model and levels are different from Lee's. Michele starts with the price of a private session ($40). The more people in a session, the cheaper it becomes. For example, a class of up to six people would pay $12 for each session. Michele also offers about a 10 percent discount for prepaying five classes or more.

List Your Prices

Once price is determined, post it on your website (if you have one) and in promotional material. If no price is listed, you may find that people call to get information and you spend a lot of time describing the program only to lose them at the price point. If they know the price up front, it saves you the time of explaining it repeatedly. If your personal training work is done on contract to corporations or local community centers and gyms, most of your negotiating on programming and pricing will be done on a case-by-case basis, and your website or promotional material will need minimal pricing information.

As part of your pricing strategy, make the payment options as simple as possible. Payment can be made directly on your website using one of many online payment companies. Of course, if you are starting out as a small and local business, the easiest solution may be to simply have clients email you directly to register and follow up with payment by electronic transfer, check, or cash. If you're concerned that you might lose track of money given to you directly, insist on electronic transfers before a program begins so that you have a confirmation on attendance, and there is no danger of losing payments.

Finally, create and explain your refund policy in clear terms. Make the policy fair to your clients as well as to your business. There will always be people who ask to circumvent your policy, and you must be prepared to stand firm and avoid treating clients differently. Establish policies that account for all situations you might encounter, each program type you offer, and all client groups you work with. On the FAQ page of her website, Lee has a refund policy stating the following terms:

> *WoW Power Waking is a small business. We try to help you out as much as possible while ensuring that we stay in business to serve you in the future! If you registered for a program and need to cancel before the program has started, we are happy to refund you in full. If the program has started and you have to withdraw for any reason, we cannot offer a refund. Please be aware that missed classes can be made up at other classes during the time frame of the session for which you registered.*

Identify Your Audience

Whether you are working in an institutional fitness environment or from within a small wellness business or are a committed personal trainer or avid walker, you could have a range of people interested in walking. In all those situations, you might find people who have never exercised before for whom walking has an accessibility appeal, or you may have people who are active in other ways and would like to try something new and low impact. These could be people of all ages, fitness experience, injury, and health history. You can create a successful walking workout program designed to accommodate a broad range of demographics and paces.

Keep in mind that different groups or individuals may have different reasons for their interest in walking. Some may like strength, flexibility, or balance exercises included in a walking program. You may find others who want to walk in a local race or fund-raising event; you could design a Six Weeks to Your First 5K program to meet their needs. As much as a walking class suits a range of demographics, you might have good success targeting a specific group to ensure that you offer what they want. For example, you might have different walking groups for new moms, seniors, those with joint replacement, or those who walk for weight loss. See chapter 9 for more details on how to accommodate everyone in your walking programs.

Set the Schedule

Now that you have an idea of who will be walking with you, consider what would work for them from a scheduling point of view. Be sure to plan for the future: first class, first program, half year, year. Think of yourself, too. Can you commit to teaching at this time and on this day on an ongoing basis throughout the year?

Time

Outdoor walking classes can work at just about any time of day, although early morning and evening classes may mean that you will be walking in darkness. Walking without daylight means special requirements for clothing and location to ensure safety for your participants. For example, walkers should wear reflective clothing (see chapter 8 for more detail) and the area should have good lighting.

Timing, like pricing, can be tricky. Knowledge of your audience is essential. If your target audience is young parents, consider a morning or lunch class when children will be in school. If potential clients live in a community with a high proportion of commuters, you may have better luck with early morning or after-work classes that accommodate the commute time. Early morning classes for people who work must be scheduled to allow people time to go home, clean up, eat breakfast, and travel to work. Likewise, evening classes for working people must be scheduled in a way that accounts for your clients' ability to get home, change clothes, and enjoy a quick bite to eat.

If you offer classes in a corporate environment, early morning (especially if showers and changing rooms are available) can help your participants to avoid rush-hour traffic by arriving at work early for walking fun. Lunchtime classes work well, too. Similarly, if you have a location close to many places of business, set a time that is within 45 to 60 minutes of 5:00 pm, the typical end of day. That allows enough time for people to change and get to you, yet not so much time that they want to go home first. Always consider how your participants will get to class and leave time for that. If your walkers are driving to class, make sure that there is parking.

Frequency

The frequency of your classes is also an important consideration. We know that typical physical activity recommendations suggest engaging in activity five times a week for at least 30 minutes. You may not have the option or interest to offer five classes, particularly not at a specific time that would work for everyone. Consider having a few options that would get people out at least twice a week. For example, consider early or midmorning sessions on Monday, Wednesday, and Friday and lunch or evening sessions on Tuesdays and Thursdays. Remind participants that taking a day between high-intensity classes to recover from the workout helps their bodies to get stronger and faster. Other activities and just general daily movement should be advised between workouts. Quite often, early morning, midmorning, lunch, and evening weekday classes can be offered along with one weekend class. Saturday and Sunday mornings are typically available for a range of demographics.

Seasonal Considerations

Plan for the change of seasons in advance. Spring is a good time to start programs in some climates because people are excited to get outside after winter. Fall is also popular, because people look forward to getting back to a routine after summer vacation. Even for outdoor walking programs, January is a good time to begin programs to coincide with the annual enthusiasm for New Year's resolutions. Many people who register for January walking programs stay with you the whole year because very little about weather discourages them. Extremes in your environment such as severe cold in winter or high heat and humidity in summer should not be reasons to stop your walk program, but you will want to make adjustments. For

Session-Based or Event-Specific Schedules

Coaching Tip

For almost two decades, Lee has offered 8-week sessions of classes throughout the year. Typically, two 8-week sessions combine nicely to create a 16-week session that is seasonally based. Three 16-week sessions cover 48 weeks of classes over the year through the winter, spring-summer, and fall season, leaving time for a two-week summer vacation and a two-week holiday break in December. You may have other priorities for setting a schedule. For example, Michele's classes are often tied to specific events since she tends to partner with other organizations.

example, if snow falls, you may need to relocate to an area that is plowed regularly. You may enjoy moving into a local mall if weather conditions pose too great a risk for your demographic. Snow and ice can make walking treacherous, but the cold can be managed by apparel change. High heat and humidity can be accommodated by changes to both class scheduling and drill organization (see chapter 8 on seasonal considerations).

Throughout the year, holidays, celebrations, and campaigns provide opportunities to organize special walks around a theme for marketing purposes, to give back to the community, or to just have fun. Here are some to get you started.

- *January*—New Year's Day, Martin Luther King Jr. Day
- *February*—Heart month (www.heart.org and www.heartandstroke.ca), Groundhog Day, the Oscars
- *March*—National Shoe the World Day (March 15, donate shoes to those who need them https://soles4souls.org), the first day of spring
- *April*—National Walking Day (first Wednesday); Walk to Work Day (first Friday); World Health Day; Walk at Lunch Day, Opening Day for Trails (www.railstotrails.org), National Park Week, Earth Day (April 22)
- *May*—Physical Fitness Month, Stroke Awareness Month (www.stroke.org); National Arthritis Awareness Month (www.arthritis.org, www.arthritis.ca); National Physical Education and Sports Week; National Senior Health and Fitness Day (last Wednesday)
- *June*—Alzheimer's and Brain Awareness Month (www.alz.org), first day of Summer (longest day of the year)
- *July*—National Father–Daughter Take a Walk Day (July 7), National Simplicity Day (July 12, walking advocate Henry David Thoreau's birthday: Slow down, step into nature, and enjoy simple things like a walk)
- *August*—National Tell a Joke Day (August 16, bring a joke to walking class), National I Love My Feet Day (August 17)
- *September*—National Women's Health and Fitness Day (www.fitness-day.com), first day of fall
- *October*—Walk to School Day (www.walkbiketoschool.org), ADHD Awareness Month (www.adhdawarenessmonth.org, www.caddra.ca, www.caddac.ca)
- *November*—American Diabetes Month (www.diabetes.org, www.diabetes.ca), National Buy Nothing Day (day after Thanksgiving, a good day for a walk instead of shopping)
- *December*—National Sock Day (December 4, take your favorite socks for a walk), first day of winter

Arrange the Location

Consider the conditions that make a program safe and fun while knowing your legal responsibility for permits. When planning your walking workout classes, evaluate your environment for safety and logistics to reduce barriers to attendance. Urban, suburban, rural, and indoor environments each have advantages and challenges. Before you finalize a location, walk the area on the days and times that you plan to hold class so that you are familiar with potentially dangerous situations and find places for walking drills. Consider how many people you can manage in the environment. Safety is your top priority. In all environments, participants should be encouraged (if not required) to wear reflective apparel or lights during early morning and evening classes in darkness (see chapter 8 for more detail).

We've had quite a bit of experience in scouting out good locations for walking. For the past six years, we've presented walking workouts at the annual ACSM Health & Fitness Summit. Each year, the location is different and presents new logistical and environmental obstacles: high humidity and multiple lanes of traffic in Orlando, hot temperatures and both pedestrian and vehicle traffic in Phoenix, a conference center hotel surrounded by highways in San Diego, and cold temperatures and a somewhat sterile corporate landscape in Arlington.

Before we arrive at the summit, we scout the area by virtually mapping it using Google Maps' satellite view to hunt for parks or trails to accommodate groups of 40 to 60 people. Once onsite, we walk the area to determine the best location, keeping in mind that we have only an hour for the session, and we cannot take more than 10 minutes to reach a suitable location for drills. We see what is available within that radius of the conference center to find the best location possible. We also do our best to walk the routes the day before our session at the times when our sessions will be held.

For regular classes, we have a lot more flexibility, but we've made these conference situations work by being creative. We've held our classes in parks that aren't much more than pathways from one block to another, in outdoor shopping areas before they open, around the perimeter of a sports stadium, and as a last resort, in parking lots or roadways of the event's hotel or conference center. Sometimes, we've even had to use different locations depending upon the time of day. We hope this inspires you to be creative with your walking classes.

Permits

Once you identify a suitable place to hold a walking program, check in with authorities, such as your local recreation department, conservation authority, or local government office to determine if you need a permit to hold an outdoor walking class. Laws and regulations can vary from one municipality to the next, so do your homework. For instance, you may not be charged for walking on sidewalks in some cities and towns, but others may restrict commercial operations anywhere on public streets. Under these circumstances, you may find that you can work with a local recreation center, a library, museum or heritage society, or a conservation area as an alternative. In parks, restrictions may be more likely. In contrast to more traditional fitness classes, walking workout classes are, by their very nature, on the move. You can be flexible about the route you take, so be clear with authorities about the exact details of what you are doing. Clarify that you can make last-minute changes to your route that will not disrupt park conditions and activities.

Small groups that are stationary may need permits because you may be occupying a specific area. If you know that you need a space (for example, you want to stay in one place for a strength training component for 30 minutes after walking), you will need to reserve it. Municipalities may not have any formal guidelines or experience working with these types of programs and may be hesitant to give it a try. If you run into resistance or concerns, a helpful resource may be the American Council on Exercise *Guide for Policymakers and Fitness Professionals on Shared Use*. You can find it on their website at www.acefitness.org.

Facilities

Most people want access to toilets before and after the walk, and possibly during. Find a location where these facilities will be open during your class time and during the season you are holding the program. Some public restrooms close seasonally. Another concern your participants may have is their ability to store things like purses and briefcases. This will be especially true in urban environments when they are coming to class from work via public transportation. Consider collaborating with a local business such as a fitness apparel or shoe store, a coffee shop, or café so that participants can leave personal belongings in a safe place at these businesses. In suburban and rural locations, participants usually drive to class and can leave possessions in their locked cars. For those participants, you'll also want to choose a location where parking is available and, preferably, free.

Sharing Your Outdoor Walking Space

Outdoor fitness groups have become more popular in recent years. It makes sense since it feels good to be outside. When leading these programs, aside from following legal regulations for any permits or business licenses, be mindful that you are sharing the space with the general population. Use common sense and good etiquette as you lead groups outside. Consider the following respectful practices.

- Choose areas and times that are less busy to minimize interference with pedestrian, cycling, or vehicular traffic.
- Be friendly and respectful to people you encounter while you are outdoors. Your interaction may inspire them to join you in the future.

- Keep noise to an appropriate volume for the location and time of day.
- Stay on the right when walking on sidewalks, paths, and trails, always leaving room for oncoming and passing pedestrians.
- Treat any infrastructure, such as benches, railings, and landscaping, with respect.
- Leave no evidence of activity.
- Participate in and encourage participation of your clients with organizations that are building and improving local outdoor space to support physical activity.
- Be familiar with any safety hazards and know how to access medical help.
- Be insured for potential accidents. (See the Insure Your Business section earlier in this chapter.)
- Educate your participants as to these best practices.

Urban

In the city, high population density means that you have a better chance of attracting more participants to your class. However, that density means more cars and bicycles that can pose serious threats to pedestrians. Even pedestrian congestion can make interval training a challenge.

Safety in the City

Cities vary in their commitment to pedestrian safety. If you live in a city where sidewalks are well maintained, free from obstruction, and not overly crowded, then a walking class should work well. Have guidelines in place for walking workouts on busy city sidewalks. Participants must

- always cross at intersections,
- not cross on yellow lights,
- stay as a group (think about the maximum number of people you could manage at an urban intersection and limit your class to that number) while crossing intersections as much as possible, and
- wear reflective clothing or gear and lights during early morning and evening classes.

Note that cars making right turns at intersections are a particular hazard for pedestrians. Drivers often pull up to intersections looking left for cars coming from that direction on the perpendicular crossroad, without checking to the right for pedestrians who may be crossing the road. This common danger is exacerbated in cities where right turns are allowed on red lights.

Class Logistics

In many cities, it is better to meet in parks where trails (paved or unpaved) are available, vehicles are restricted, and the environment is conducive to having large groups of people participating in walking workouts. Even small parks can work if you use your creativity. Shorten speed drill timing and use benches, curbs, and other structures, like you might in larger parks for strength intervals, practicing balance, or as landmarks for speed drills. Tiny "pocket parks" in high-density cities can be used as time-outs for the dynamic warm-up, strength exercise segments, and a cool-down. These small corners of quiet are perfect for describing your drills to participants before doing them. For example, tell them to walk alternating city blocks: Walk one block fast, do squats while waiting at the corner for the rest of the group, and then walk one block more slowly for recovery. This is a good way to keep the group together, especially so that people cross intersections as a group. Also, this strategy avoids needing to shout or use a whistle over urban noise to manage the workout.

Lee coaches in Toronto, and she offers evening and early morning classes on city sidewalks. Evening can be trickier than early morning because sidewalks are busier. For both times, it has worked well to search out quieter residential streets, school tracks, college grounds with green space, and paved trails in ravines (for which Toronto is famous).

Suburban

Like urban areas, suburban areas offer good population from which to draw an audience for your workouts. Usually, there is less vehicular traffic, wider roads, and sidewalks, making both safety and class logistics a little easier to manage than in city areas. Sometimes outdoor mall complexes might be available to you at off-peak hours. With lighting, bathrooms, and in some cases music, they can be very appealing, especially in the winter since the sidewalks are always clear. If you are considering this as an option, speak to mall management.

Safety in the Burbs

Suburban areas have varying commitments to pedestrian safety. It is probably fair to say that most suburbs were designed for vehicles. Roads are wide, and while there are sidewalks, intersections can still be large and dangerous. If stoplights are present, they often have short pedestrian crossing times. In some towns and suburbs, there may be no sidewalks at all. When this is the case, it is common practice to walk on the side of the road facing oncoming traffic so that you can see what's coming. We recommend this only if the shoulder on the road is wide and you have a small group of no more than five people. If you do this, be aware that you'll need to change sides of the road, walking with traffic, when going up hills or around curves. In these situations, drivers coming up a hill or heading into a bend will see you sooner than those going in the opposite direction. You want drivers to spot you with enough time to react. As soon as you crest the hill or round the bend, cross the road so that you're walking against the traffic again. On winding roads, you may end up changing sides frequently. No matter what side you're on, always be alert, and remember: If you can't see a car coming, the driver can't see you either.

Similarly, even in quiet neighborhoods, on flat roads, a large group approaching an intersection may be faced with a car making a quick right turn from a side road position that is out of sight to the group. Given the propensity of so many drivers to look to the left while approaching intersections, many drivers see oncoming walkers only after making the turn and leave themselves no time to stop or move away from walkers.

If you use a looping technique (see chapter 5) to get faster walkers to return to the larger group, it is essential that they cross the road to face oncoming traffic as they loop. It may be necessary to consistently remind people to never turn their backs on traffic except in the hill and curve scenario described above.

In general, locations without sidewalks or paths should be considered only if there is a wide shoulder and if you have a small group. Otherwise, the risk for accidents is just too high, and the program will suffer in quality.

Class Logistics

Though designed for cars, suburban areas typically offer more green spaces and quieter residential areas for walking classes. Staying in residential areas allows people to spread out over longer intervals. Cul-de-sacs and small residential blocks offer good locations for beat-the-clock drills (see chapter 5). If your class is held early in the morning, you may have large, empty parking lots accessible to you. The painted lines of empty parking lots can be used for speed and technique drills, allowing people to practice "walking the line" (plank) to encourage the development of hip rotation technique (see chapter 4). Schoolyards offer structures for strength drills and tracks for speed work. If your class participants have great variations in pace, tracks keep everyone in one place and in sight. Keep in mind that there are always class participants who find track work tedious. Consider starting and finishing at a location that allows you to walk through trails or pleasant residential streets to get to the school and do just a few drills at the track. Or, do track workouts on alternate days to keep things interesting. If you use a track or other circular path, change the direction in which everyone is walking halfway through your session. This will ensure that people do both left and right turns for a more balanced workout and body.

Rural

The beauty and quiet of rural locations make for inspiring walking. Despite the low density and reduced traffic, the lack of sidewalk infrastructure makes safety and class logistics challenging.

Safety in the Country

The greatest danger of walking on rural roads is that drivers are not expecting pedestrians and are often moving at a high speed. Another factor to consider is the distance from help should anyone take ill or fall during class. Walk in areas that have cell service, always carry your phone, and have a strategy in case of emergency. For example, have a first aid kit on hand, know whom you might send for help, carry emergency contact information for all participants, and have a plan to get the rest of the class back to the start location. Knowing your participants' health histories is absolutely critical. For example, should any participant have prediabetes or diabetes, have some sugar tucked away with you on walks. Encourage, or make mandatory, bright clothing at all times. The more visible you are to motorists, the more time they have to react to your presence on the road and the safer you and your group will be.

Class Logistics

Even the smallest of towns usually has a local school with a track, or at the very least, a place for people to park their cars. There may be a park or green space that features trails or walking routes. While it may be difficult to do speed drills on uneven trails, hills can be used for incline repeats to create a cardiorespiratory workout, even one that includes HIIT (see chapter 5). A short length of paved trail or sidewalk can be used for speed intervals. Roads that do not service a lot of trucks can be used. The rules that apply to suburban walking in the previous section also apply here. Always walk facing traffic and encourage people to stay on the shoulder and off the main road. Be especially mindful climbing hills, looking for oncoming vehicles that cannot be seen until they have crested the peak. Watch for cars making a right turn from a crossroad that could put them directly into your path. Keep in mind that unpaved shoulders of rural roads make for slow walking. Whenever you must walk on uneven surfaces, encourage good form and remind participants that the workout will challenge leg muscles in a different way than paved roads.

Indoors

It may be that outdoor walking is limited where you live for all or some of the year. Alternatives that may appeal to you include mall walking and treadmill classes.

Safety Inside

Mall walking is typically safe from traffic and air-quality concerns as well as hot and cold weather challenges. Still, most mall floors are made of concrete or other hard surfaces, which may lead to foot issues such as plantar fasciitis. Encourage your participants to change the terrain underfoot for some of their personal walks if your class takes place indoors. Their shoes may need more cushioning to manage the hard surface and possibly more lateral support depending on the size of the mall. A small mall will force walkers into frequent and tight radius turns, necessitating more lateral support than when walking outdoors. Also, as noted earlier, make sure that people change the direction in which they walk so that left and right turns are balanced. This is also something to keep in mind if you hold your outdoor classes on a track or similar circular paths.

Treadmill walking offers the same protection from traffic, air-quality, and weather concerns as mall walking without the concerns for lateral movement overuse and hardness of surface. Your most important safety consideration is ensuring everyone knows how to use the treadmill, especially how to safely start and stop. When they are changing the speed or incline, remind them to do so slowly to allow the machine to catch up, otherwise they may adjust their speed or incline too high. Also have participants check that their shoelaces are secure and short to avoid getting caught in the belt. Encourage focus. Distracted walking can mean that your participants are pulled backward off the treadmill.

Class Logistics

Most mall walking can happen only before store opening hours. This may restrict you, or it may invite a regular crowd! You'll definitely have to ask the property managers if it is something you could offer. They may charge a fee, and you will probably have to show proof of insurance.

Treadmill classes require that you find a venue with treadmills. From a logistical point of view, this might be more challenging than starting outdoor programs. Still, it's worth considering, especially if you already work at a gym with treadmills. It's a workout that could be sold to runners as an excellent form of cross-training and even a way to improve running technique in that they can learn shorter stride, faster cadence, and powering from the arms. Alternatively, you could lead this class for both walkers and runners because treadmill classes easily accommodate people with a wide range of paces without having to worry about keeping them together as is necessary in outdoor classes.

While the focus of this book is face-to-face training, you may find that a client wants to work with you, and it is impossible to schedule that time. You might end up coaching someone online or over the phone if they are highly motivated to get out the door on their own but want ideas on how to increase the challenge. Before you begin, make sure that you know as much as possible about where they walk, physical health, and goals. Ask questions about the conditions under which they will be walking. Be sure to make safety recommendations related to their location, whether urban, suburban, rural, or indoor environment. It's a good idea to ask them to send you short videos of their walking technique to ensure that form will not lead to injury.

Keep good track of your notes and your weekly recommendations for workouts. Try to balance coaching on form and speed. You can recommend interval workouts, especially ones that include self-compete drills (see chapter 5).

It's All in the Details

For many coaches, their strength is programming, including class content, motivation, and people. The administrative side of operating a business or group can bog them down. If you are this person, ask or pay someone to help you. If this is not possible, especially if you are a small business and need to keep costs low by doing administrative tasks yourself, create a schedule to manage specific tasks, and stick to it. See appendix C for an example of the tasks you may want to schedule on a regular basis. Here are suggestions for how to manage the most common tasks.

Attendance

Keeping track of who is coming to class can be helpful in sustaining the program over the long term. Create an attendance sheet, either paper or electronic. If you have a smartphone, you can fill it out right away. There are also a few apps created for taking attendance. You may find one that you enjoy using. If a person signs up for a weekly class and misses two classes in a row, that means you have not seen them for three weeks! It's time to touch base. Follow up with an email. People can be embarrassed to return to class after an absence. When you send them a quick note, it encourages them to return.

Email Management

Do you have 7,000 emails stored on your computer? Time to clean up! Receiving, replying to, and creating emails can consume an extraordinary amount of your administrative time.

- *Receiving*—Set up separate mailboxes or folders within your email server account in which you can file emails according to subject matter or even class registrations. You may even be able to set it up so that incoming messages are automatically filed, organized, and distributed. For example, if you offer online payment and registration, all those emails would get placed into a separate inbox so that you always know who has registered and paid for your classes.
- *Replying*—Many people set aside specific time each day to reply to emails. Ideally, emails from clients or potential clients should be answered within 24 hours. If you have a query button on your website, make sure that the emails that arrive via that option have a designated mailbox or folder so that you can reply quickly.
- *Sending*—Any time you create an email, ask yourself if the email is serving its intended purpose. Does it need to be sent at all? Would a quick text or phone call be a better choice? Ensure that you follow good email etiquette in terms of the message recipient list (cc and bcc). Almost always, the right thing to do when sending an email to a group is to put the addresses on a bcc list. Unless individual clients have specifically given you permission to share their email and you need people to reply-all, the bcc email etiquette works well.

Delegate When Appropriate

If you discover in the first few months that the key administrative tasks described previously are not getting done, or are not getting done effectively, consider hiring someone to handle them for you. Advancements in online technology have made it easy to find good help, including virtual assistants. These assistants, who can be especially helpful for small businesses, can help with repetitive tasks such as keeping attendance and payment records, sending health forms and waivers, collating health forms and waivers, writing weekly or monthly emails or newsletters, bookkeeping, and more. While you may feel this eats into your revenue, your ability to use your strengths where they are most valuable will help you build better programs and be the best coach, which will lead to more clients and a more successful business.

Growth of Your Business

As you and your participants settle in to your walking workouts, give attention to encouraging and managing growth. The most successful business owners not only adapt to change but also welcome and plan for it. Growth and change can take many forms, as we'll explore here.

Coaches

Even as an independent personal trainer or avid walker starting with a simple plan to introduce just one or two walking classes each week, you should think about who could lead these classes in the event you take a vacation or have a personal emergency. This person could come from within your walking group or, if you are a personal trainer or group fitness leader, you may have a colleague who has expressed interest in leading walking workouts. Invite any substitute coaches to attend a class or two to familiarize themselves with your class format. At a minimum, a substitute leader needs the confidence to lead a group and an understanding of the components of the workout, including the warm-up, drills, and the cool-down. Also, anyone who leads the class should have current training in CPR.

Thinking even further ahead, nurture the relationship with substitute coaches by encouraging them to gain a fitness certification (if they don't already have one) and to become a regular coach for you. If your groups are growing (more than 15 to 20 participants), consider using an assistant coach. You could split the group in two for drills or simply have the assistant stay at the back of the group to ensure no one gets left behind. You might discover that you want to permanently create two groups, and this assistant could take over one of the groups.

Support Staff

We have talked about keeping on top of the administrative side of your walking program. If you want to grow, this work will become more demanding. Some of the previous suggestions will become essential to expansion. If you have been doing everything yourself, invest in support for three key positions that will free up a lot of your time: a bookkeeper, an accountant, and a web support person.

More Classes

If you find that classes are consistently pulling in more than 25 people, it's time to add more classes to the weekly schedule. Also, if you notice that your walking workouts are the only cardiorespiratory exercise that people are doing, it's a good idea to offer three or four of them a week at accessible times so that people can attend at least two of those classes each week. If participants are doing three or more classes a week, they will notice great improvement in cardiorespiratory fitness, and it may reduce risk for injury. Participating in just one class a week and not doing other forms of physical activity or walking regularly outside of class leaves muscles, tendons, and ligaments vulnerable because of the contrast between so much inactivity and intense activity.

Specialized Walking Classes

You might be surprised to find that your program draws a high percentage of people new to exercise because walking is an accessible form of exercise that appeals to many who never enjoyed going to a gym or participating in formal exercise classes. For these people, walking classes that include a strength component is valuable and desirable. You've probably gained their trust and can suggest several new forms of movement and classes to them, including walking boot camp, marathon walking, walking and strength, walking and stretch, and mindful walking.

Having gained their trust as a coach, you may discover that clients are eager to try classes you offer that have no walking component at all. These might include hiking, stand-up paddleboard, outdoor yoga or stretch, outdoor strength, Pilates, tai chi, or even roller blading.

Stay Creative and Fresh

You need to keep things fresh for your business. While your walking drills may stay rooted in the same principle of interval training over the years, there are a number of ways to change the experience for your participants from one workout to the next. Sometimes all it requires is taking a few minutes to sit and imagine how you could tweak the timing, change the location, change up drill order, find new cues or analogies, or bring in current research. The resources that follow may fuel your creativity.

Attend Conferences

Just as the face-to-face experience of walking class is so powerful, attending conferences to meet other professionals and hear experts speak remains one of the best ways to stay inspired and motivated as a walking coach. So much research on exercise physiology, anatomy, nutrition, mindfulness, coaching techniques, behavior change, and more is relevant to you and your participants. Take it back to them. We attend ACSM's Health & Fitness Summit, canfitpro's World Fitness Expo (in Canada), and the biennial National Walking Summit put on by America Walks.

Walk to Find Inspiration

Coaching Tip

Michele created a new walking workout one day when she didn't feel like walking. She managed to get out the door by setting a goal of one mile at a leisurely pace. She averaged a 19-minute-per-mile pace. By the end of the first mile, her mood was improving, so she went another mile a little faster, averaging a 17-minute-per-mile pace. Feeling even more invigorated and happy, she picked it up to a good brisk pace, coming in around a 14-minute mile. For the final mile, it was a race to see how fast she could complete it—11.5 minutes! Four miles were completed on a day when she didn't feel like walking. She has used this same workout with private clients in person or virtually, and it's a great way to boost motivation and finish with a sense of accomplishment.

Read

Stay current by reading material that is both focused and wide-ranging. Many magazines and books have information pertinent to your work as a coach. These could come from the fitness industry, including publications focused on walking, running, and strength training. You might also broaden your learning to include books that cover human endurance, mindfulness, the environment, and the human condition. The list is truly endless. See the list of recommended reading in appendix A.

Walk

We wager that your most powerful ideas will come to you when you are taking your own walks. Stanford researchers found that creativity increases up to 60 percent when people are walking compared to sitting [1]. Experiment with drills. Explore new routes. Let your mind wander. Play with both body and mind. Insert boot-camp-style strength or plyometric drills. Use different mantras or cues to walk faster. Let the power of walking circle back to you, helping you become the most creative and inspirational coach you can be.

With your plan for walking classes and programming in place and a strategy for growth, you are ready to promote your classes and the concept of walking as a workout. In the next chapter, we'll look at best practices for getting the word out and people walking.

References

1. Oppezzo, M. and Schwartz, D.L. 2014. "Give Your Ideas Some Legs: The Positive Effect of Walking on Creative Thinking." *Journal of Experimental Psychology* 40 (4): 1142-52. www.apa.org/pubs/journals/releases/xlm-a0036577.pdf.

11

Promote Walking as a Workout

Ongoing communication builds loyalty. The key is to use the many tools at your disposal to communicate to current and potential walkers. From social media posts to emails and e-newsletters, all have a role in building your walking community. The following sections offer many ideas about how to promote your walking programs.

While they might be considered traditional, methods such as writing articles for local papers and fitness newsletters can also be very effective in letting people know what you do and what you offer. Send news releases to local papers with stories about your new walking program. If you have client success stories, include them in the press release, but secure permission from your clients first. In many communities, walking workout classes are a novelty.

Social Media

Nearly 66 percent of American adults and 75 percent of Internet users belong to social network sites such as Facebook, Twitter, Instagram, and Snapchat. Success in social media can mean success for your business or program. Or, social media can suck all your spare time! Know your demographic. If they are not using a specific social media, or any at all, you'll get little return on your investment in time. If they are using it, a smart social media strategy will enhance your connection to them and may grow your audience as each platform has an ability to advertise your programs.

Live streaming on social media platforms is becoming more popular and is more accessible to users than reading blogs or written posts. It is particularly suited to promoting walking. You can take your phone with you on a walk. You can talk about walking technique. You could video drills as they happen in your class. It's worthwhile to search recommendations on effective live streaming because it is a skill to be behind or in front of a camera!

Positive messaging across your social media platforms is necessary. We will emphasize positive language in the next chapter on coaching, but choosing positive words in all communication, whether verbal or in print, works to build energy. Humor can be effective in person but problematic online if it includes any negative word choices. For example, sarcastic humor is difficult to pull off effectively in person and impossible on social media. Before sending a message out on social media, reread it for tone and energy as much as for spelling errors.

Finally, always search for any new trends on social media. Use them to enhance your ability to inspire, encourage, and promote walking. For example, know how to follow and use hashtags (see the #Walking section later in this chapter).

Facebook

Most businesses have a Facebook page because it is the most accessible social media platform to a wide demographic. For clients who use Facebook, it can be a timely and effective way to communicate and motivate, especially if posts are a mix of inspiration, information, and promotion. We both have business pages separate from our personal Facebook pages and highly recommend it. Facebook offers a place to post your contact information, including physical location, website, and phone number. Post photos and videos to keep your followers engaged. The frequency of posts depends on your goals and resources. Facebook can also be used to schedule and advertise special events. Perhaps you plan on holding a casual but timed 5K walk to introduce walkers to races. Facebook allows you to set up the event with a description, time and day, and an option to promote outside of your own followers. Be sure to create events for each of your classes. If you decide to boost one of your posts in the form of an ad, the possibilities to choose your budget and your audience (including location and interests) are highly effective.

You could even set up special groups within your Facebook page. Perhaps a group of walkers is interested in meeting up for social walks on their own? Maybe people are interested in setting a distance goal over a month or a year? They can walk on their own but post to the Facebook group about their progress. As an administrator of such a group, you can help them stay motivated, and they will do some of the motivating, too! If you find that negative comments are being posted, you may want to consider setting up the group in a way that requires you to authorize all comments before they are visible to the entire group. If this becomes too time-consuming, ask one of the members to take on the role of approving posts.

Twitter

Twitter has turned out to be a powerful platform for spreading and learning about current events. Its claim to fame is brevity. No post or tweet can be longer than 280 characters. This brevity is somewhat deceiving, given that any tweet can embed a link to a website, article, photo, or video. This has made it the go-to platform for getting the latest news and research. As a coach, you may find it valuable to follow reputable experts in walking, exercise, and nutrition. The information they post could be shared with your participants.

If your participants are on Twitter and following you, a simple retweet shares that information with them. Otherwise, you can share via email, newsletter, blog post, or other social media channels.

You may want your Twitter feed, as well as your other social media accounts, to be entirely related to walking. Or, you may want it to be more personal and include walking. It is easy to create separate Twitter accounts each with its own focus—something you may want to consider for Instagram as well. Large corporations, small businesses, academics, celebrities, and individuals all use Twitter.

Instagram

The fact that every Instagram post is either a photo or a video makes it inherently appealing and well suited to promoting fitness and a healthy lifestyle. It can be a positive and empowering online space. On the other hand, it can turn into a narcissistic display of unrealistically fit bodies. Research has shown that photos of selfies and perfect bodies invite self-comparison, discouragement, and even shaming [1]. We personally have found that photos of beautiful outdoor spaces that you can imagine yourself walking in are much more inspiring.

If you have your phone with you during class, taking quick photos of some of the walking class fun can be inspiring to post on your Instagram page. Typically posting once a day or every other day will inspire without inducing fatigue or boredom. Care should always be taken to take photos of people from behind or the side in a way that they are not easily recognizable, unless you have written permission to post images of them on social media. Sensitivity to the privacy of your clients is paramount.

Having said that, Instagram has a feature for direct messaging. This allows you to send photos to specific groups without broadcasting to all your followers. This may be a helpful feature if you'd like to post a group photo that includes recognizable faces. Still, it's good policy to ask everyone if they agree to the photo being broadcast to the group. You can also do this in releases that participants sign before joining classes.

Snapchat

Snapchat allows you to send video content to followers. More than 70 percent of Snapchat users are between the ages of 18 and 34. It is very possible if this is your demographic. However, the latest polls suggest that Snapchat is losing favor even with young people, so check in with your clients before investing time in this platform.

Social media platforms can be an easy and fast way to set up a walking group or business because they are inexpensive and a simple way to connect people. Here are suggestions for how to get started using these platforms.

- Create and post a short video or photos that inspire people to join your walking workout.

#Walking

Using hashtags on social media can help to grow your walking business or programs. A hashtag is any combination of words put together without spaces and preceded by the pound sign (#). Hashtags are used to categorize information posted on social media and to make that information discoverable by others. About 75 percent of people on social media use hashtags. Here are 10 essential points to help you use hashtags to your advantage.

1. Hashtags are created and managed by users; that means *you.* Create your own hashtag or use ones that have already been used. On Twitter, hashtags link your tweet to a conversation. On Instagram, they describe content in your post. On Facebook, hashtags work best on an open business account rather than a personal account with security privacy settings.
2. Using appropriate hashtags can help you draw followers and interest in your walking business or programs.
3. For your hashtags to get traction, your social media accounts must be public; otherwise, only people who are already following you will see them.
4. Hashtags can be used on Instagram and Facebook stories by using the hashtag sticker or simply inserting the hashtag into the text.
5. Hashtags are most effective when they are specific to the content of your post. For example, #walking as opposed to #niceday, or #intervalwalking versus #health.
6. Based on research, the number of hashtags that are most effective varies by account. For Twitter and Facebook, it is one or two hashtags; on Instagram, it is 8 to 10. Hashtags on Instagram can be inserted into the comment section to keep your caption clean.
7. Use hashtags that are appropriate to your current audience and potential audience. To tap into the correct audience, consider checking out hashtags of your competitors (such as local fitness businesses) and do searches on social media using hashtags that you think might be relevant, such as #walk, #walking, #speedwalking, #powerwalking
8. If you post with a popular hashtag, your content may get missed because there are so many other posts under this hashtag, but it also has the potential to go viral because of the wider audience.
9. A hashtag that has few followers may reveal a niche market for you and potential branding opportunity. Experiment creating different hashtags and reviewing the response.
10. In addition to creating and using hashtags on your own posts, follow hashtags to stay up to date on trending information.

- Use hashtags to promote your videos and posts on social media platforms. Though each platform uses hashtags a little differently, popular hashtags for walking include #powerwalk #powerwalking #speedwalking #walkworkout #outdoorfitness #(name of your town) #outdoorfitness. Add these hashtags to any post you make.
- Follow up any social media posts with more social media posts!

Website

Websites are today's storefronts. Even if you have an actual storefront, your website is probably where people will go to learn more about your programs. Think of it as your first opportunity to greet and inspire. When people arrive at your website, let them be inspired by who you are and what you are offering. Give them a sense of your authenticity, integrity, and excellence. This can be reflected in photos and words. Show visitors what you value: photos of where you walk, what you've seen, and maybe where you plan to go. There might be photos of groups walking together to show that you appreciate community. Tell your story, and post quotes that speak to you. You can find inspiration and ideas on the Internet under subjects such as inspirational, motivational, funny, nature, and positive.

The information on your website needs to be updated consistently. Good design invites people to stay on your web page and sign up for your program. Essential information that must be readily accessible after landing on your home page include your business name, information about you as a coach, contact information, and a list of your programs, including time, date, duration, cost, and registration details. Use photos to maximum advantage: smiling faces, people walking, outdoor beauty.

Websites have become easier to design and implement in the past decade, making them less of a financial burden to create and maintain. If you need assistance creating your website, you can find a wealth of accessible information on the Internet regarding set up and design or ask small-business owners you know to share their website creation experience and suggestions. You may want to consider hiring a web assistant. Still, you, as the visionary, should always visit your website on a regular basis with an observer's eye. Check out every page to ensure content is current and accurate.

Photos

If you have photos posted on your website (and we hope you do!), ensure that they match the current season. It doesn't work nearly as well to solicit participants for summer classes with winter photos on your website. Ensure that any waiver you send out to participants has a disclaimer allowing participant photos to be used on your website or anywhere else you might want to use them such as social media. See examples of waivers in appendix B.

Class Descriptions

A website can look out of date quickly if your courses are posted when they are long completed. Courses should be removed from the website before they are finished so that you can post upcoming sessions. Leave a note that drop-in classes are available at any time. Try to have your next session of classes posted at least four weeks in advance so that people can plan. If you offer special annual workshops or events, try to post them at least two to four months in advance. If an annual event is popular, post the time, date, and fee for the next year as soon as possible after each event concludes.

FAQs

You will quickly discover that many people have the same questions about your program. It is helpful to answer these in advance on your website. This should be reviewed and updated annually or whenever any key information changes.

Here are suggested questions that you may want to post and answer on your website to save yourself many hours on the phone or email.

- What is power walking?
- Is power walking racewalking?
- Is all the walking done outside?
- What if I have not exercised in a long time?
- What should I wear?
- What should I bring?
- Is there a place to leave my things?
- Is there a restroom?
- How do I know which class is best for me?
- Do you offer refunds?

Payment Buttons

If you are taking payment online, payment buttons need to be created for each course session on the online payment website. Once registration for a course is full or the course is over, be sure to delete these payment buttons from both your website and the online payment website through which you process your payments. This prevents clients from being able to access old payment buttons at old prices because they have not cleared the cache on their computers.

About You

Newcomers often visit the About page on your website. Refresh it annually with a new photo of you and your coaches. While you're in there, update your descriptions and bios. You'd be amazed what changes in a year.

If you write a blog, update it on a regular basis so that your audience knows when to expect it and you appear engaged in your business. A better option may be to write a regular newsletter to people who have requested to be on the distribution list.

Newsletters

Small-business experts have differing opinions on newsletters. Some see it as junk mail that clutters inboxes and ends up mostly in the trash. Others view it as a valuable way to offer your clients or group participants added value with tips and inspiration as well as information about upcoming programs. Choosing an appropriate frequency and including meaningful content will go a long way to making sure that your newsletters are read and not just sent to trash. If your sessions operate on a six- or eight-week basis, you can use newsletters just ahead of the start of new sessions to generate registrations.

Create a goal connected to your newsletter that is consistent with the needs of your audience. If you're simply trying to sell your classes, people will stop reading them or cancel their subscriptions. Include good information that offers people value without cost and be sure that this information is either within your scope of practice or includes references to experts. Examples include walking tips, information about local walking events, nutrition advice, strength and stretch guidance, fitness and wellness research, and anything that is inspirational.

If you create an effective newsletter, it will become an anticipated arrival to inboxes. Include photos to make it visually attractive. Post it to your website so that visitors to the site can find what's current with your walking business. Maintain an archive of newsletters on your website, and regularly confirm that it is current with your most recent newsletter.

The most popular tools for creating newsletters include Mailchimp, Campaign Monitor, and Squarespace. The template design, editing, scheduling, and tracking abilities of these online software programs make them a powerful tool for communication. Most have a no-fee option as well as upgrade options that typically offer more precise scheduling and data collection. Even some no-fee options offer valuable information, including tracking who is opening the mail, the number of clicks on embedded links, and simultaneous posting to Twitter and Facebook. If you don't already have an e-newsletter, check out some of these options. Most of them offer tutorials on how to maximize their power.

There is a business case against sending out e-newsletters, especially if you already send out a weekly email to class participants and are a regular user of social media. Many of us already receive too many newsletters and delete them automatically as they arrive. Still, we have found that most registrations for classes happen after a newsletter has been sent out. Experiment for yourself. You will soon learn what gets you the most feedback for your effort.

Emails

A weekly email to people currently attending your walking classes is one of the best ways to encourage consistent attendance. Remind them of the time and location of the next class, make suggestions for what to wear based on weather forecasts, or list upcoming local races that they might be interested in walking. You may also want to offer a quick tip on walking or nutrition (if that is in your scope of practice). Just keep it short, and people will be more likely to read it. Always review any information given out in these emails vocally during the beginning or end of class for those who may have missed it or didn't have time to read it.

Lee has found that a weekly email to clients works well for her business. She sends out an email on Monday mornings to participants currently registered in classes and a few longtime clients who have asked to stay on the distribution group. The email includes information pertinent to the upcoming week, including a reminder of days and times for classes, weather forecasts, parking, or travel logistics (such as road or public transit closures). It acknowledges participants who completed walk races or events over the past weekend. Sometimes advance notice is given of special events—for example, a special workshop or walk. If you send emails, include links back to your website and social media platforms as well.

Texting

An alternative to email may be texts. Michele has found that her walkers tend to prefer getting class reminders and information via text. They also then use texts to update the group on how they're doing and offer support to each other. It has even led to group members meeting up on their own to walk. This works well with small groups, but it could be unwieldy and disruptive with larger ones. If you want to text a group, always get permission from everyone first since you'll be sharing their phone numbers.

Texts are also a great way to quickly get in touch with individuals, for example if you're expecting someone at class but they are late. You could text them to check in

Word of Mouth

Recommendations from people who know you, and especially people who have taken your classes, are the best way to recruit people to join your walking program. You could offer an incentive, such as a gift card to a local coffee shop or a discount for walking classes, that will inspire people to spread the word. Or just ask them to do it. It is amazing how willing people are to give you a positive testimonial when they trust you, value your coaching, and want your program to be a success.

Advertising

You may discover, as we have, that advertising can be expensive relative to your revenues. Traditional advertising media may work, but much of it is considered antiquated and costly. Lee had some success in the early stages by putting ads into local newspapers but later found that it was more helpful to use social media, even paying for broad distribution of posts and events. Still, the old-fashioned strategy of posting flyers, especially in the immediate area of your program location, can be low cost and effective. Be sure to have the time, date, cost, and length of your walking program. Consider including a short bio of your coaching, walking, and fitness experience. Photos, according to conventional sales wisdom, boost readership, so have great photos of the places you will walk.

Ask for Feedback

Honest feedback is invaluable to your walking business. A simple survey sent out via email is an easy way to collect input when you have small class sizes. As your class size (12+ participants) or frequency (3+ classes per week) increases, consider using a more formal survey approach such as that offered by an email marketing app. These apps allow you to easily track response data in a report format.

Questions for the Walking Coach

If you are the sole coach, answer the following questions to help you identify if the program is working for you. If you manage another coach, ask them to give you written answers (or use a survey tool if you have multiple coaches) to these questions so you can review and respond as appropriate.

- Do participants feel safe in class? Do you feel safe?
- Did you meet the goal set for number of participants?
- Is the walking location easy to manage?
- Are you able to manage the pacing of the group effectively?
- Do classes finish on time?
- Did everyone pay promptly?
- Is your payment system easy to manage?
- Are you able to manage attendance accurately?
- Do you get at least a few minutes to speak to each participant during each class?

Questions for the Participant

Using the following questions, or others that are important to you, ask for written comments or simply a score on a scale of 1 to 10. Ask concise questions, and not too many, to encourage people to answer them. You may want to add specific questions at times; for example, you might ask participants if they would like to add strength exercises to a class if it's not already offered.

- Do you feel safe in walking class?
- Do you enjoy the location(s)?
- Is the class what you expected?
- Do you get a good workout?
- How would you rate the exertion level? Easy? Hard? Just right?
- How would you rate your energy before class?
- How would you rate your energy after class?
- How would you rate your mood before class?
- How would you rate your mood after class?

As you gather input about your walking classes, keep in mind that it is impossible to make everyone happy all the time. Address any areas of concerns or dissatisfaction as best you can, especially any safety considerations that may come to light. Use the feedback to confirm what you're doing is working and identify areas of improvement that could make your business even more successful.

Get Involved in Your Community

There are so many factors in our society that decrease opportunity to experience meaningful face-to-face time with people. The resulting isolation adversely affects health. Humans need human interaction. Your walking classes offer an antidote—creating a community in which people get out of their offices and houses, step away from their computers and cell phones, share stories, and support each other in achievement. The logistics of walking class allows participants to get to know each other. During the warm-ups and cool-downs and between speed drills, there is time to chat and build camaraderie. Face-to-face time is critical to building trust and human relationships. You are offering a powerful service in the creation of this human community, and this will build loyalty to your business.

This effect will be compounded when you encourage and participate in your extended community. It will help grow your business and provide a profound sense of belonging to you and your participants as well as to your community. In many cities around the world, the first weekend in May sees many Jane's Walks. These are walks in honor of Jane Jacobs, an urban visionary. Consider offering a free walk that focuses on fitness, and you might find that you recruit regulars to your program. Create a walking team for a local cleanup day. Wear matching shirts that feature your logo. Promote any campaigns or celebrations that align with your emphasis on

StoryWalk

Case Study

Some kids no longer have to choose between reading a good book and playing outside. Instead, they can walk or run outside while reading a story. StoryWalk features laminated pages of a children's book attached to stakes that are erected along a walking path or hiking trail. As children and their parents walk (or run) along the route, they can read the story.

The concept was created in 2007 by Anne Ferguson of Montpelier, Vermont. At the time, Anne was working as a chronic disease prevention specialist and wanted to design something "different, fun, and interesting" that would get parents and children to be active. "Active parents have active children and physical activity is a key component to chronic disease prevention," says Anne.

After researching copyright issues, Anne posted the pages of David Ezra Stein's book *Leaves* along a popular path in her local park and included a notebook for feedback. The response was overwhelmingly positive, and the program grew throughout Vermont, into all 50 states, and into 14 countries with the help of Kellogg-Hubbard Library in Montpelier. The program is entirely funded by public donations.

Many StoryWalks have been set up by libraries, but they can be done by anyone or any organization that's interested. They can also be set up around schools or community buildings or in store windows in downtown areas or shopping complexes. Indoor locations such as museums, hospitals, schools, community centers, or assisted living facilities are other possible venues. Books with more text or less text could be used, and pages could be spaced farther or closer together, depending upon the audience's physical abilities. Some children's groups have even written and illustrated their own stories to post.

For more information, go to www.kellogghubbard.org/storywalk.

walking or physical activity in general. (See the monthly marketing ideas in the Seasonal Considerations section of chapter 10.)

Here are more ways you can get involved in communitywide initiatives.

Races

Even the smallest communities offer fund-raising walking events and races. Encourage your participants to enter and train for them or volunteer to staff a water station or aid station at a local race. Get to know the race organizers and tell them that you train people to walk for fitness. Ask them if they offer a walk category and if not, encourage them to do so. There may be opportunities to work together on creating a walk division (see chapter 8, The Race Case to Support Walking Divisions). Fundraise for their event if it's a cause you value.

Community Walkability

In many large cities across North America, there is a growing awareness that the walkability of neighborhoods is vital to human and community health. Walkability is broadly defined as an ability to walk with ease in an area as made possible by things like good sidewalks, lighting at night, buffer zones between pedestrians and cars, landscaping, crosswalks, and removal of obstructions such as lamp and utility poles. Even in smaller towns, there is growing recognition that pedestrian accessibility and safety is paramount to long-term health.

You can be a change maker in this area. Share your understanding of how physical activity is one of the most important ways to promote good health. Explain how good infrastructure, such as sidewalks, lighting, intersection design, and more improves the walking experience. Describe how walkability improves home value, lowers crime, and increases traffic into local businesses, resulting in an improved local economy, increased community satisfaction, decreased vehicular traffic, and much more. For more information on making your area more walker-friendly, check out americawalks.org.

Your own commitment to walkability has an exponentially powerful effect. As your walking business grows, your passion for walkability is shared with class participants who, in turn, will likely join you in supporting improvements to local streets. Then, as the community becomes more walkable, interest and participation in programs such as your walking workouts will increase.

Ongoing Collaborations

If you are a personal trainer or group fitness leader, it may "take a village" to help you grow. There is great power in collaboration with local organizations and businesses. Small businesses will be sympathetic to the need to work together to grow business in a complementary way. Michele has had success in marketing her walking programs at a women's weekend retreat. In exchange for offering three or four walking classes during the long weekend, Michele gets to attend the retreat and participate in all the other offerings, about a $1,500 value. Since the women aren't directly paying for the class, there's no debating over "paying to walk," which is a common obstacle to building a walking business. Once the women experience the class, they see the value, and in Michele's experience, they have then been more willing to pay for her services, often telling her that she should charge more. This venue also introduced Michele to a new demographic with more disposable income.

Local coffee shops and running stores are obvious places to check with. For example, plan a walk from a local coffee shop. They might offer a discount on beverages if you bring a group. Local running stores may be a

Discovery Walks

Coaching Tip

During a conference in a suburb of Vancouver in 2009, Lee wanted to go walking, but the neighborhood did not seem inviting. She committed to head out for at least 30 minutes to see how the neighborhood stacked up. Within 10 minutes, she found herself in front of the Richmond Olympic Oval, which was being built for the 2010 Winter Olympic Games. She walked inside and discovered a gem of a public space that would be used for the community when the Olympics were finished. From that experience, Lee decided to offer a two-month peripatetic walking class every year. *Peripatetic* means to travel from place to place so, each week, the class travels to a new location in the city, giving participants a workout and an opportunity for exploration and discovery.

good place to meet for the start and finish of your classes. They may offer their spaces for free in exchange for the possibility of business that your walkers will bring. They might also offer you a deal on shoes or clothing to purchase if you add their logo along with your logo. These businesses may let you post flyers or advertise your classes through their social media and newsletters. You might even approach other businesses, such as a wellness center, pharmacy, or clothing store, explaining how their business may benefit from supporting walking.

Community centers and libraries may allow you to post flyers and may offer you space to meet at the beginning or end of class. If you present your program as a local service, they will be more likely to support you.

Also, look for informal walking groups in your area. You may see them out walking or find groups through an online search. Individuals from these groups might join your regular classes, or the group might invite you to lead workshops.

Any promotion that you undertake will be doubly effective when word of mouth confirms that your walking workouts support your marketing claims. Since coaching makes or breaks client satisfaction, it is worth taking a closer look at how to build coaching excellence. In our next chapter, we'll examine the best practices to bring to coaching.

References

1. Tiggemann, M., and Zaccardo, M. 2015. "'Exercise to Be Fit, Not Skinny': The Effect of Fitspiration Imagery on Women's Body Image." *Body Image* 15 (9): 61-67. https://www.ncbi.nlm.nih.gov/pubmed/26176993.

12

Coach for Success

When people feel good at the end of a class, they come back. Research shows that exercise has a mood-lifting effect [1]. So, if you offer people a well-designed workout that gets them exerting themselves, they are going to feel good. With the many ways to get the heart pumping, what will make people return to your walking program and classes over other fitness programs?

A good coach and a well-coached program!

Let's explore ideas to make that happen.

What Makes a Good Coach?

The secret of any successful fitness program is a knowledgeable and motivating coach or instructor. This is especially true for walking programs since walking is something that people view as inherently easy to do on their own. We've heard this before: "Really, who needs a coach to go walking?" Or, "I already know how to walk." But few people break out of a stroll when walking on their own, let alone achieve a moderately vigorous walk. A good coach has the power to transform walking into an athletic, heart-pumping workout; build a community around walking that makes sticking to exercise easier; and inspire people to transformational change. Let's look at how you can be *that* coach.

Authenticity

A simple definition of the word *authentic* is genuine or real. What do we mean exactly when we talk about someone's authenticity? A bully can be a genuine bully, but when we describe a person as authentic or genuine, we typically mean it as a compliment. An authentic coach has integrity and lives what they coach.

Harvard Business School professor Bill George says authentic leaders have four qualities. They are people who constantly learn and grow, are able to manage their emotions to communicate effectively even in difficult situations, are willing to admit their mistakes, and are sensitive to the needs of others.

Motivate with a Streak

Coaching Tip

To keep your clients on track when they're not with you, encourage them to create streaks. A streak is where you do something every day and have a visual reminder of it. For example, they could make a construction paper chain or string of beads, adding to it each time they walk. Because no one wants to break a streak, they're motivated to push past the usual excuses of no time, too tired, or bad weather when walking on their own. If they don't walk one day, they break the streak and have to start a new chain or string. They can also do this electronically with apps such as Chains.cc, Streaks, HabitHub, and Goal Tracker & Habit List.

At the core of what George describes is a person with integrity: Someone who exhibits integrity seeks the truth, seeks to share that truth honestly, seeks to live that truth honestly, and seeks to understand and respect the truths of others. You exhibit integrity when you live by this code under all circumstances because the person you present yourself to be is the person you are. Who you are in private aligns with who you are in public. It is not changed by money, celebrity, or even whom you are talking to. This means that everyone you coach is seeing the same person.

Walk the Talk

If you want to inspire people to walk for exercise, you are going to have to enjoy doing it yourself. Only then can you find your authentic coaching voice, and your enthusiasm will be infectious. Everyone will want to walk with you and will trust your expertise. How might this play out? Let's say that your enthusiasm for walking inspires a participant in your class to register, train, and walk a 5K race. They ask you to coach them through that process. You have never walked a 5K race or coached anyone to walk a race. Give them two options rooted in authenticity. First, tell them that you have no personal experience walking a 5K race, but you are willing to help them and will educate yourself by reviewing research and talking to people with more experience about the process. You might even commit to walking one yourself to gain firsthand experience. The other option is to refer them to another coach who does have that race experience. Either way, your integrity and honesty give them permission to make a decision based on what is best for them. If they decide to work with you, it is because they trust you to be authentic and honest. If they choose to work with someone else, you can be sure that this is a positive reflection of your encouragement and confidence.

GirlTrek

Case Study

One of the biggest and most successful walking movements was conceived by two college friends, one working in education and the other in digital media, who were motivated by the health crisis that they as black women, their friends, and their families were facing. Black women die younger and at higher rates of preventable diseases than any other group of women. To encourage black women to take charge of their health, T. Morgan Dixon and Vanessa Garrison turned to an inspiring ancestor for motivation. If Harriet Tubman could walk to freedom, they could walk for better health.

So, they started walking and experiencing its benefits. Morgan took groups of students on hikes, and that's where they came up with their group's name, GirlTrek. In 2010, they asked friends and family to join them in a 10-week walking challenge and to share it with others. GirlTrek officially became a nonprofit organization in 2012. The organization is a grassroots effort that relies on volunteers to start up groups in their communities. From a few hundred women taking that first challenge, the group continues to grow with about 170,000 women at press time and has become the largest health nonprofit for black women and girls.

While many of the women have lost weight and improved health markers like blood pressure and cholesterol, GirlTrek is about more than just fitness, which may be the key to its unprecedented success in engaging black women. It's about black history, self-worth, healing bodies, inspiring daughters, and reclaiming communities.

In 2015, GirlTrek bussed 500 women from 10 cities around the country to Selma, Alabama, to participate in the 50th anniversary of the march from Selma to Montgomery for voting rights for African Americans. Those who couldn't go to Selma were challenged to complete 54 miles—the number of miles protesters marched—during the month.

They regularly challenge women to keep moving with prayer walks, Harriet Tubman walks, and other challenges inspired by their history. In May 2018, they released *Harriet's Handbook*, a self-guided, yearlong walking challenge with hundreds of ideas and walks.

Along with reclaiming their bodies and health, they're reclaiming their neighborhoods. They're cleaning up blighted areas and beautifying them. They're advocating for safer intersections and better walking conditions to encourage others to start walking. And they're not stopping. GirlTrek's goal for 2020 is to have 1 million black women and girls walking with them.

For more information, go to http://girltrek.com/.

While we tend to think of people who are coaches as people who are the very best, even champions, at whatever they are coaching, this is not a prerequisite. You do not have to be faster than all the people in your classes. Looping strategy and drill organization that keeps people in one general location allows you to manage a range of speeds, including those faster than you are. Even your walking technique does not have to be perfect. It helps if you can demonstrate all aspects of walking technique, but the most important skill is to be able to identify ways to help others achieve it.

Listening

Everyone loves to be heard. If you are a skilled and active listener, your participants will give you a high score for coaching. Asking questions is the precursor to listening! Start with a health questionnaire before participants join your program. During class, have several open-ended questions on the tip of your tongue to draw out information. *How are you doing today? How was your week? Tell me about your walks.* Listen to their answers so that you are always learning, just like your clients are. Listening is the foundation of learning. Coaching your participants to success happens when you know as much as possible about their ability to walk and their walking goals and then use that knowledge to personalize how you coach them.

Before Coaching

Even before you meet them, get to know your participants by having them fill out a health questionnaire. Until recently, a basic questionnaire for the fitness industry used to be the Physical Activity Readiness Questionnaire (PAR-Q) form. It asked seven health-related questions, and if a person answered yes to any of the questions, it was recommended that they seek medical clearance before doing any physical activity.

The PAR-Q was replaced with the Get Active Questionnaire (GAQ) and you may prefer to ask for even more information. See appendix B for details on the GAQ and other examples of questionnaires that you might use.

It is helpful to ask if they have any concerns about exercise and walking specifically. Asking an open-ended question like that can be revealing and often provides useful information for you. Another good open-ended question might be to ask if they have any specific goals as a walker. If they have no goals, encourage them to set some. This will help them see improvement through effort and gives them a tangible sense of their ability to change, which helps to keep them motivated. Follow up by asking them if they foresee any challenges to achieving their goals, and encourage them to come up with ways to overcome these obstacles when they arise. Being prepared with a plan can help them stay on track, and there's more buy-in when they participate in their own solutions.

In Class

Possibly one of the greatest rewards of leading a walking program is that you have an opportunity to get to know your participants. There is time to chat, ask questions, listen to answers, and read the unspoken emotional messages. If you lead a 60-minute walking class with high-intensity intervals that consume anywhere from 10 to 30 minutes, you will be left with 30 to 50 minutes to connect with your participants. At the beginning of class, do the math for how much time you can allot to each participant. For example, in a 60-minute class with 20 participants, you've got 3 minutes with each participant. Subtract time required to talk to the group as a whole during the warm-up and cool-down and the time for the high-intensity WPs, when you encourage a focus on effort and not talking. Make sure that you connect with each participant at least once for one question, using the ideas in the Listening section earlier in this chapter. Whatever happens, you will have connected with that participant in a meaningful way and gained valuable information. For instance, someone may confess that they've been so busy at work that they haven't walked in several days, so you'll want to make sure they get challenged in class. If you hear that someone is recovering from the flu, give them permission to take it a bit easy. Other times, you may learn more general information, perhaps a family member is dealing with a health crisis and they are worried about the future. Mentally file, or even write down, the information for later use if appropriate.

After Class

It takes very little time to follow up with a participant who needs extra attention or who has been missing from class. Sending an email or text takes just a moment. Texting might be appropriate if you were definitely expecting someone in class, and they did not show up. Email is less intrusive because our expectation is that emails do not need to be answered immediately. Consider sending an email if they have not been in class for a week or more and did not mention that they would be away. Use a subject line like "Checking in." In the body of the email, use casual wording that is free of judgment and expresses concern, such as, "We've missed you in class for a few weeks and wanted to know how you're doing. Hope to see you next week!"

Know Your Stuff

Just as you listen to your participants, keep listening to experts in the field. Stay on top of the latest research in health and fitness. Obviously, anything that specifically pertains to walking performance is important. You've made a great start by reading this book. Keep reading! Read books and magazines about walking, fitness, and health. You might learn an interesting tidbit related to walking or one that you could relate to walking. It's also helpful to read running magazines. Many drills, tips, and principles that runners use also apply to walking. If your participants are interested in competing in races as walkers, running magazines have many helpful ideas. Go to conferences to learn about the latest trends and research. Follow known experts on social media, especially Twitter, making sure that you check their credentials. Look for scientists doing research on topics like exercise physiology, exercise psychology, biomechanics, exercise science, nutrition, walking, and running at accredited universities. You might find excellent fitness professionals to follow by going to conferences. Always check certification status and research experience. There are also excellent journalists who report on research and trends.

Watch for any topic that may help you bring something of value to the table as a coach, including guidelines on physical activity and nutrition, athletic performance, mental health, apparel, and motivational tools. You may not be an expert, and even if what you learned is outside your scope of practice there are ways that you can use it to help your clients while staying within your scope of practice. For example, if someone is noticeably dragging in class and they identify fatigue as an issue, you could ask if anything has changed for them in the past week or month. Maybe they are trying a new diet in which they are eating no carbohydrates. Your query may help them connect the dots between their change in diet to fatigue. That might be the perfect invitation to explain that you know from your reading that carbohydrates act as fuel for the body during vigorous exercise. You do not need to tell them to eat carbs, but just by explaining the role of carbohydrates, you might get them to figure out what they need to do to avoid fatigue the next time they come to class. The more you know about anything that can affect the physical and mental health of your participants, the more you bring authentic, authoritative leadership to your role as coach.

Know What You Don't Know

Truly understanding what you do not know and being honest about it is absolutely essential to becoming an authentic coach. It speaks to your integrity and makes any advice you offer clients meaningful. They will come to respect that any recommendations you offer are based on both knowledge and experience. They will trust that you have been transparent about any possible gap in your knowledge.

This does not mean that you must stay quiet unless you are absolutely certain of information or can cite scientific research. It simply means that you identify the reliability of any information or advice you offer. For example, you may say that you read about a good exercise to prevent plantar fasciitis in a reputable running magazine, and it helped several walkers you have trained. Another example might involve identifying a specific food as being high in magnesium, if someone is asking about foods that are a good source of electrolytes. Remind them you are not a registered dietitian, and offer reliable sources for them to follow up with their own research. You can help by identifying information as common knowledge, as a topic that researchers are currently studying, as

What Is a Physiatrist?

A physiatrist could be the answer when you or your client have a stubborn condition. This type of doctor specializes in physical medicine and rehabilitation with the goal of getting you back to doing what you love with the least invasive treatment as possible. They often treat people with pain, muscle or bone injuries, or nerve damage that affects movement or quality of life. When Michele was sidelined with foot pain, she saw a podiatrist and an orthopedic surgeon without getting any relief. It was finally a physiatrist who connected the dots—weaknesses in her hips were resulting in the foot pain and strengthening that area corrected the problem.

anecdotal evidence from personal or client experience, or as a controversial idea that may require further research. The key is to be upfront about your information sources and to present any information in a way that is not prescriptive.

Knowing what you don't know also means knowing when to refer your clients to specialists who can help them with specific issues beyond your scope of practice. While it is good to know several in your area, it is not a prerequisite to making a referral. Simply knowing the type of professional who might best suit your client's concern can be valuable. Some of these health specialties include podiatrist, physiatrist (see previous section What Is a Physiatrist?), massage therapist, orthopedic, sports medicine doctor, psychologist, registered dietitian, life coach, naturopathic doctor, or physical therapist.

Adapt Your Programming

Be mindful of the response you get from people in classes. Your ability to be attentive to how participants react to your programming and class structure will play a vital role in ensuring their success as walkers and your success as a coach. Perhaps your demographic is largely comprised of stay-at-home parents. Morning classes scheduled between school drop-off and pick-up is one way of showing that you are listening to their needs. Moving the start time of summer classes to an earlier hour is a great response to participants saying that they do not enjoy walking in the heat. Perhaps you've heard complaints that a walking location is too noisy and busy, suggesting that it's time to consider a move to a quieter location. Listen to any ideas that come up about programming. Someone might say that it would be nice to include strength training in the program. Try offering a walking circuit for six weeks. Are registrations dropping when you make a change? Send out an email asking for feedback on the change, keeping in mind that you will not be able to please everyone all the time and that you are still the exercise expert.

During class, are you watching people's facial expressions and body language? Grim faces, slumping bodies, and shuffling feet are signs that you've pushed too hard. Find a way to let them recover and recharge. Tell a joke or point out something of beauty. Perhaps the opposite is happening. Everyone is happily chatting, and the intensity of their effort is not enough to challenge them. It's time to find your motivational voice and get them going. One surefire chat stopper is to have them count their steps during an interval (see Counting Steps drill in chapter 5). They can't talk while they count, though some may try. You might hear half-hearted complaints, but everyone will be happy for the push. They are in class to be challenged; otherwise they could be walking and talking on their own without a coach!

Speaking

Being comfortable speaking and giving direction to a group of people is a requirement of leading outdoor walking classes. Your voice should be at a sufficiently loud volume to be heard, and it should project authority so that people respond to direction. If your voice is not naturally loud, it can still be authoritative.

There's nothing like a whistle to bring authority to instruction. Always have a whistle with you and create a specific whistle protocol. For example, one whistle blow means speed interval begins, two whistle blows mean recover from the speed interval, and three whistle blows mean loop and return to the coach (see chapter 5, Learn to Loop).

Exuberant extroversion, especially if it is not your authentic personality, is not a requirement for inspiring coaching, but other speaking skills can turn you from a good coach into a great coach.

Positive Language

It seems obvious that you want to project positivity as a coach. Encouragement goes a long way to getting the best from people. High-fives and compliments build feel-good energy and self-esteem. Compliments that focus on effort are especially helpful. In her book *Mindset: The New Psychology of Success*, Stanford psychologist Carol Dweck describes how coaches encourage a growth mindset in their clients when they reward effort over specific performance data such as pace or finish times. In her words, "people with a growth mindset . . . admire effort, for no matter what your ability is, effort is what ignites ability and turns it into accomplishment." In walking class, this means recognizing when someone is attending class consistently and putting effort into the conditioning segment of the workout in such a way that interval times are improving. Let them know that you are noticing this effort. It goes a long way to reinforce continued effort. As an aside, this is why benchmark walks work so well to reveal the positive effects of effort.

Another strategy that brings an encouraging vibe to class is to find the positive version of all instructions. For example, find a way around the word *don't* as much as possible. If you are leading people through a hamstring stretch that involves placing one foot at an elevation and hinging the torso forward at the hip to access the stretch, a common error is to fold at the waist trying to get the upper body closer to the thigh. The temptation is to say, "Don't fold at the waist" or "Don't round the back." Instead, visualize what you are trying to achieve in terms of body position to maximize the stretch and say those words. In this case, say, "Hinge at the hips, keep the rib cage high, and pull the hip away from the heel. Visualize a line from the tailbone to the crown of the head." Keep in mind that while you want to keep it positive, sometimes comparisons between the right way and wrong way to do an exercise can help clients to get it. In this hamstring example, you could suggest participants round their backs and notice if they feel any diminishment in the stretch happening in the hamstrings.

Another example might happen during the conditioning segment of class. You are instructing people to set out on a speed interval, walking as fast as possible until they arrive at the next street corner. Suggest that they loop back to you. Ask them to keep moving. Avoid saying "Don't cross the street" or "Don't stop." The trick to doing this successfully is to

My Pleasure!

It is common to hear people reply *no problem* to the words *thank you*. We believe it is more powerful, and joyful, to reply with *you're welcome, my pleasure*, or a variation on those positive responses. First, replying with *no problem* implies that the situation could have been construed as problematic, which may not have been the case at all. Secondly, we diminish our role as coaches when we temper our response to the gratitude that is being expressed toward our work. Using positive words as much as possible creates an environment of success and empowerment for coach and participant.

constantly ask yourself how to use precise and specific words to create a positive visualization. The challenge of this effort will be worth it, and the more you do it, the easier it becomes. It's a subtle way to bring a positive energy to each moment in every class.

In the same way, avoid *yet, however*, and *but*. Many people have learned to offer a compliment before a critique, and that is good policy. It's made even better when the positive statement is not followed by any of those three words. Obviously, your job as coach will involve critique. The trick is to use positive language and presentation to do this. For example, it would be typical say to a participant, "Kathy, your arms were working well in that last interval, *but* remember to keep your eyes looking to the horizon." Instead, try something like this: "Kathy, your arms were working well in that last interval. You can enhance that power by keeping a tall posture with the eyes looking to the horizon."

Humor

It's been said that laughter is the best medicine, and we agree. In a 2018 study published in the journal *Psychology of Sport and Exercise*, researchers found that the oxygen cost of running was less when smiling. In other words, smiling made running easier [2]. Though they did not study power walkers, it's reasonable to think the result would be similar.

Even if smiling doesn't make running or walking easier, we do know that seeing someone smile makes us smile back. Smiling feels good. Try it out right now. If you are smiling when you are coaching, your participants will smile back. Lee loves organizing drills in such a way that two teams can walk in opposing directions. As they cross paths, she encourages them to "high-five" each other, which always results in smiles!

Other ways to engage people in humor include getting them to "strike a pose" between intervals. Or, "power pose" before they start intervals. When doing chalk drills, encourage people to express their inner artists. Simply bringing a sense of play to class gives participants the opportunity to smile and laugh so they'll look forward to coming back.

Succinct Cues

We've all had the teacher or coach who just talks too much. While stories can be engaging and powerful in elucidating what you are trying to get across, fewer words while coaching are often most effective. Using succinct language means people can keep moving because it is not necessary for them to stop to listen to you. It's especially effective when people are putting maximal effort into a drill, and they need silence to concentrate. Yes, silence is golden. A few short words could help them visualize their strength and speed. *Stand tall! Pump the arms! Let's go! Dig deep!* Use a tone in which they can hear the exclamation marks and keep it to just one or two cues per interval.

Set Your Boundaries

Walking classes offer a valuable opportunity to chat, allowing you to get to know your clients and your clients to know each other. It's a time when you can share your walking stories. This creates a camaraderie with your students and a powerful, positive energy in the class. Remember that it's important to know when you've talked enough.

You should set clear boundaries in your mind. For example, you may talk about your family but always keep any information about them positive. When considering the stories you tell, ask yourself if the subject of your story would feel comfortable walking beside you as you are telling it. If not, it's not appropriate to share in your class. Likewise, protect any information that participants tell you in private, especially if it is health related. If you are saying inappropriate things, you are disrespecting the person about whom you are speaking. Anyone listening will wonder if you will treat information they tell you in a similar manner.

It's also a skill to know when the talking needs to stop. Sometimes group conversations may bring a cloudy mood to class. This is especially true if a tragedy is overwhelming the newscasts or a political situation is getting tense. People will bring this into class. It can be good to let everyone get concern out of their systems. Your class is not a bubble floating separate from the real world, and to deny people emotional support and caring is unrealistic. Be patient with the group conversation but have an exit strategy in place, such as bringing people back to the task at hand. Set them up for a stretch or a drill. It is also reasonable to restrict certain divisive topics like politics and religion during class to maintain a sense of unity. Know how to change the subject. Intervals work well for this purpose!

Another aspect of setting your boundaries as a coach is to avoid extending your reach into a client's life a little too far. You will learn a lot about people when you walk with them. You will know when they are ill, when they are going through emotional or financial trouble, or when their children or spouses have upset them. You can be a good listener, and you can show respect for how these things affect their training and their well-being, but your responsibility ends there. If, in your professional opinion, they need help, it is reasonable to refer them to community resources. Keep a list of these handy for quick reference when situations arise.

Similarly, you will need to be authentic about any difficulties in your own life without creating drama around it. We all go through difficult times. You can be honest about the situation without drawing them in or making them feel obligated to help you. You are still the coach.

Always Know Your Primary Coaching Objectives

Every time you develop a session or lead a class, embark on the task knowing what you want to accomplish. You may find it helps to communicate your objective to class participants. When they understand why you are doing something, they are more likely to embrace your plan.

Define the Program

Class sessions that run six to eight weeks tap into the well-known physiological ability of the body to change in that time. Anything shorter than six weeks, and people are unlikely to experience noticeable changes. Anything longer than eight weeks, and they may lose a sense of commitment or sense of purpose. Consider having specific goals over those weeks. For example, while you always want to maintain conditioning, you may emphasize hiking as part of one session to improve proprioception. Or introduce a series of three or four strength exercises during one walking session, such as push-ups, lunges, or planks, to add a measurable activity to the workout that reinforces how physical effort results in physical improvement.

Plan Each Class

The first goal for any class is to begin and end on time. This is one of the most basic ways to show respect for your participants. It helps to have a method to communicate with anyone who may be arriving slightly late to class. For example, suggest they text or call as soon as they know they might be late. You can reply with the direction the group will be walking. You can do a walk loop partway through the warm-up to meet them. It is rarely helpful to wait for people to begin. This can become a habit and dramatically reduces the enjoyment for participants who have showed up on time. For the coach, arriving 10 minutes early for class is arriving on time. Likewise, ending the class on time shows respect for participants' time. Assume everyone has somewhere to go after class, even if it's for coffee!

When you arrive at class, have a plan in mind. For example, your warm-up will be a 10-minute stroll, followed by dynamic warm-up exercises in a small park. Then, along a short path in the park, you'll do a series of 8 go-recover intervals for 30-seconds each and 6 beat-the-clock drills from 45 to 60 seconds each. You'll finish with walking lunges, a stroll back to your starting point, and 10 minutes of stretching. Always check in with

> ## Unplug
>
> ### Coaching Tip
>
> A great coach uses the cell phone only when needed: for a class emergency or before class has started to let a participant who is late know the direction you will be walking. Otherwise, cell phones should be tucked away in silent mode. This is true even if you are alone before class waiting for people to arrive. Be ready with a smile for your first participant to arrive.

that plan at the halfway point in class. Make sure that you can make it back to your start or end location on time. If not, make any changes necessary to do so. It's better to arrive at your finish destination a bit early and insert strength exercises or extra stretches than to arrive late.

Manage Individual Objectives in a Group Setting

Your plan for any class or program will have to work with the objectives of individuals in the class. This is a balancing act. There may be walkers who regularly enjoy walking half marathons. They will have different needs and coaching requirements than participants who are there for a self-contained workout. It can be tempting to show extra attention to the person who is training for races or the person who is always asking questions. Ask yourself if you are meeting the needs of individuals in a way that does not leave other participants feeling sidelined. Ultimately, your objective is to lead an energizing and motivating class. If one person in that group verbally indicates that their needs are not being met, consider suggesting personalized one-to-one coaching. Or, perhaps a different program taught by another coach whom you believe would be a better fit.

What Makes a Well-Coached Program?

As much as your motivating, knowledgeable, and empathetic coaching will engage participants, your program must support and enhance your coaching excellence. Create a safe, challenging, and fun environment, and along with your skilled and enthusiastic coaching, you will be rewarded with a successful walking program.

Safety

Your priority for participants should be their safety. Always be prepared to cancel class, change a planned route, shorten class, or modify in whatever way necessary to make your walkers feel and be safe. This may require offering repeated and specific instructions for looping so they are not turning their backs to traffic. It may involve insisting that people wear reflective gear and lights to evening classes. You, too, should be following those rules. When your participants see that you are taking safety seriously, you set an example of professionalism.

Always carry a whistle, and make sure that everyone knows the signal to return to the coach. We use three whistles for that purpose. You can use it when the class is spreading out too much or to get people to come back to you when you feel a situation is unsafe, such as when walking on residential roads and walkers spread out across the whole road. Call them back for a quick reminder about staying to one side of the road.

Challenge

After you are sure everyone is safe, challenging your participants to appropriately higher levels of exertion than they would do on their own is your next priority. Earlier chapters have given you the tools to do this. Always keep it at the top of your mind when planning your classes. Even if you have to shorten a class for weather concerns, make sure that there is time for vigorous walking and ideally at least a few minutes of maximal effort. The best way to do this is by offering a few self-compete drills in every class after everyone has warmed up properly so that they are capable of this maximal effort in a safe way.

Fun

People who join your walking class are choosing to spend their limited leisure time with you. When you add a sense of play and joy to the workout, it brings a secret ingredient that keeps them returning. Here are a few suggestions to get you started and spur your imagination to create many more.

Team Creation and Naming

Separating your walking group into two groups can be fun. The easiest way to do this is to have two team names. They could be seasonally related. For example, the snow and ice teams, or the crocus and daffodil teams. The teams could be apparel related. For example, the shoe team and the sock team, the hat team and the cap team. You get the idea. Here are two fun drills that can use teams to great effect.

1. Find a small area around which two teams can walk in opposite directions. Elementary schools often have tracks that are smaller than competition tracks, but even standard 400-meter tracks can be used. Look for small grassy areas in residential cul-de-sacs or in parks. Have the teams head off in different directions. One team is walking counterclockwise while the other team is walking clockwise. You stand at the start line for both teams. They have their backs to each other at the start line because they are walking in opposite directions. Start both teams off at the same moment you begin timing. Each person walks as fast as possible around the designated route. Time them as they walk this circle, reading their times out loud as they

Using Tech to Track and Motivate

Many people find that tracking and mapping their walks improves their accountability to personal goals, inspiring them to get active, stay active, and commit to more challenging fitness goals. Here are several ways to help your clients use technology to stay motivated.

Basic Watches

Any watch with a second hand can be used to challenge walkers with intensity interval drills. If you set a specific distance on flat ground or up a hill, you can walk that distance several times measuring the time it takes to walk that distance using the second hand. It's a fun and easy way for people to push themselves to HIIT on their own. There are also watches with a chronograph mode that would make the timing easier than using a second hand. Another helpful mode is one in which two different interval times can be set. (There are also apps to do this.) For example, Lee uses this mode to set two intervals alternating 30 seconds with 45 seconds. She walks as fast as she can, counting her steps during the 30-second interval and then will recover walk for 45 seconds. (See Counting Steps drill in chapter 5.) During one walk each week, she walks these two intervals repeated 8 to 10 times.

Smartphones and Watches

Not too long ago, the pedometer was the product of choice for tracking activity. But now fitness trackers are on our cell phones as apps and on more parts of our bodies as watches, rings, and headbands, along with the more traditional clip-on option. They're tracking more than just steps, and new methods of tracking, such as through clothing, glasses, and even implants under the skin, are in development. The increase in popularity may be attributed to the greater variety of data collected that helps people live a healthy lifestyle in a more comprehensive way than simply counting steps. Trackers now have the capability to set intensity and pacing goals as well as to share data with

(continued)

return. After a recovery, have them walk that same route, trying to finish in a faster time but also giving a high-five to each member of the team walking in the opposite direction. Inserting the high-five gives them an extra time challenge on the route. And, as mentioned earlier, something about the high-five brings out a smile in everyone. Have them walk that loop three to five times or more, depending on how long it takes, and then have both teams change directions. *Note*: Before leaving on their loops, each team will need to be given instructions on which side of the path or track to walk and which hand they are using for the high-five. Otherwise, it turns into a mess of people potentially crashing into each other.

2. Hill training provides another opportunity for fun with teams. Have one team start at the bottom of the hill. Have the other team start at the top of the hill. Blow a whistle to start both teams. The team going downhill has

USING TECH TO TRACK AND MOTIVATE *(continued)*

others to create friendly competition. Research shows that users are sticking with trackers for longer now than in recent years [3].

Many specialized watches offer global positioning systems (GPS), allowing people to map their walks and track data that may be of interest, including distance walked, pace, elevation climbed, and heart rate. These watches may offer alarms that make it easy to set up timed intervals for high-intensity bursts of speed. Also, the data in these specialty watches can be downloaded to home computers for long-term tracking and greater analysis. If you coach people individually, this feature can be a great tool helping you structure and monitor client workouts—especially if you work with them remotely. Many phone apps will track everything a watch-style GPS will: mileage, pace, heart rate, and more. Typically, these apps offer a minimum service option for no cost and premium versions for a fee. A watch with GPS and data tracking is easier to use than these phone apps, but the cost is usually higher. Michele and Lee use the MapMyRun or MapMyWalk apps that store walking routes and track such data as elevation, pace, and overall time and distance.

Since many clients may already have tracking devices either on their smartwatches or smartphones, you could collaborate with your walking clients on setting goals with these devices.

Many phone apps are free, some have a cost, and some are free for minimal tracking service with additional fees for upgraded services. When purchasing wearable technology considerations beyond price point include style (many are now designed for the fashion conscious), display (ease of visibility and amount of data), compatibility to phones and computers at home or the office, battery life, and water resistance.

With rapid innovation in this area, you should check out reviews on popular third-party websites, such as www.cnet.com, www.consumerreports.com, www.pcmag.com, and www.tomsguide.com.

two jobs. One is to find their best downhill form, and the second is to shout out encouragement to the group walking uphill. The team going uphill has one job: to walk as fast as possible to the top of the hill. Both teams get a chance to walk around in recovery mode on flat ground before doing the drill again. Each team will alternate going uphill and downhill. At the end, teams walk a high-five or handshake line, just like they do in professional sports.

Lotteries

Lotteries work because people are motivated by prizes! Prize value is irrelevant; just the idea of winning brings a sense of play to the class or program. Here are two ways Lee has used lotteries in her program and classes.

1. In 2012, she challenged people to walk 1,248 miles (2012 km) over the year. It was a significant challenge that meant walking 104 miles (168 km) each month. At the end of every month, people who had committed to

participating in the challenge would submit their mileage. Each person who completed the monthly goal would have their name written on a ticket that went into a storage vault (an empty peanut butter pail) for the grand prize drawing at the end of 2012. So, if a person reached their walking commitment each month, they would have 12 tickets in the drawing at the end of the year. The prize at the end of 2012 was a four-month all-class pass to the 2013 walking program.

2. Over the summer, when attendance can be lower because people are on vacation and more self-motivated to walk on their own because the weather is nice, Lee holds a once-a-week coffee lottery in class. Before class begins, each participant chooses a folded piece of paper from a bag and tucks it away in a pocket. One of the pieces of paper is marked as the coffee winner. The other papers have fun messages suggesting that they "play again" next week. At various points during the class, such as before or after each interval, participants exchange papers without looking at them. Every time an exchange is made, someone may be giving away or receiving the winning paper. During the cool-down, participants open the piece of folded paper that they were last given to reveal a winner!

Field Trips

If variety is limited within a two- to five-mile radius of your usual starting point, take field trips. You could offer an entire four- to eight-week session that meets at a different location each week. Or, change location three to four times in a year. In summer, trek along trails or roads that are difficult to navigate in winter. This also works in an urban or suburban environment in which you may want to walk through different neighborhoods. It can even work in a rural environment where everyone meets in a neighboring town for a few walk workouts each year. Another idea is to take a field trip simply from your regular start location: Choose a destination a little farther than the typical distance you cover in class. Rather than linger in one place doing interval drills, do drills the entire way to the destination and the entire way back. For example, set out to see an amazing holiday light display in the winter or a beautiful garden in the summer.

Storytelling

Sharing stories is a powerful way to build connection among participants. This camaraderie brings a sense of fun to class. Good times for conversation are during the warm-up, between intervals, and during the cool-down. As a coach, you can encourage this by listening to stories, telling your own stories, and even mentioning the stories of participants to the group if you know you have their permission. As we mentioned earlier, there is always the possibility that one of your participants brings a list of complaints or negative news to class and use our tried-and-true method to change the topic of conversation: Begin a set of high-intensity drills, where people are counting steps instead of talking. Counting steps is a favorite!

Another way to create connections and build community is by encouraging your participants to get to know each other. For example, have a middle name day: After each interval, have people exchange their middle name with one other class participant. Repeat this after each interval so that everyone has learned the middle name of everyone else in the group. As an alternative, participants could share nicknames, favorite food, favorite movie, or favorite book.

Themes

Bringing a theme to your program or classes works well to change class routine. As you know, change is good for the body and maintains interest in the program. The Olympic Games are a fun time to role-play. Before starting an interval, ask each participant to visualize themselves as one of their favorite athletes in the Games and tap into that mindset of all-out effort during intervals. Role-playing also works during sports playoffs.

The theme of "exploration" also brings change to class. If you usually walk in a park with paved paths, spend time exploring trails. The workout might not be as intense because you cannot get the same speed on an unpaved path as on a paved path. However, it is empowering when you take people literally "off the beaten path." In urban or suburban areas, take roads you've never been on. If you happen upon a dead-end, use it as an opportunity to walk as fast as possible to the end. A dead-end makes a good landmark when doing fartlek intervals.

Perhaps you offer walks during a full moon, or winter or summer solstice walks. Bring chalk and play hopscotch as a cool-down. Bring hula hoops for a fun way to make core work part of the cool-down. Wear Santa (or other themed) hats; they make people feel good. The possibilities are unlimited.

Taking your coaching and programming to a new level of excellence will ensure that everything you have learned throughout this book about walking mechanics, fast walking, interval walk training, complementary stretching and strength exercises, managing logistics, weather and special populations, and promoting and marketing of walking workouts will make you a leader for fitness walking.

References

1. Miller, J.C., and Krizan, Z. 2016. "Walking Facilitates Positive Affect (Even When Expecting the Opposite)." *Emotion* 16 (5): 775-85. www.ncbi.nlm.nih.gov/pubmed/27100368.
2. Brick, N.E., McElhinney, M.J., and Metcalfe, R.S. 2018. "The Effects of Facial Expression and Relaxation Cues on Movement Economy, Physiology, and Perceptual Responses During Running." *Psychology of Sport and Exercise* 34: 20-28. www.sciencedirect.com/science/article/pii/S1469029217303461.
3. Patel, M.S., Foschini, L., Kurtzman, G.W., Zhu, J., Wang, W., Rareshide, C.A.L., and Zbikowski, S.M. 2017. "Using Wearable Devices and Smartphones to Track Physical Activity: Initial Activation, Sustained Use, and Step Counts Across Sociodemographic Characteristics in a National Sample." *Annals of Internal Medicine* 167 (10): 755-57. www.ncbi.nlm.nih.gov/pubmed/28973116.

APPENDIX A

Recommended Reading

Walking-Fitness Specific

Meyers, C. 2007. *Walking: A Complete Guide to the Complete Exercise*. New York, NY: Ballantine Books.

Stanten, M. 2017. *Walk Your Way to Better Health*. Emmaus, PA: Rodale, Inc.

Stanten, M. 2010. *Walk Off Weight*. Emmaus, PA: Rodale, Inc.

Fenton, M. 2007. *The Complete Guide to Walking: for health, weight loss and fitness*. Guilford, CT: The Lyon Press.

Iknoian, T. 1998. *Walking Fast*. Champaign, IL: Human Kinetics.

McGovern, D. 2016. *The Complete Guide to Marathon Walking*. Brattleboro, VT: Echo Point Books & Media.

General Fitness

Ratey, J. 2013 *Spark: The Revolutionary New Science of Exercise and the Brain*. Boston, MA: Little, Brown & Co.

Gibala, M. 2017. *The One Minute Workout, Science Shows a Way to Get Fit that's Smarter, Faster, Shorter*. New York, NY: Avery Publishing.

McGill, S. 2015. *The Back Mechanic: The Step by Step McGill Method to Fix Back Pain*. Ontario, Canada: BackFitPro, Inc.

Noakes, T. 2002. *The Lore of Running*. 4th ed. Champaign, IL: Human Kinetics.

Segar, M. *No Sweat: How the Simple Science of Motivation Can Bring You a Lifetime of Fitness*. New York, NY: AMACOM Books.

Dweck, C.S. 2007. *Mindset: The New Psychology of Success, How We Can Learn to Fulfill Our Potential*. New York, NY: Ballantine Books.

Walking Inspirational

Solnit, R. 2001. *Wanderlust: A History of Walking*. New York, NY: Penguin Books.

Nicholson, G. 2008. *The Lost Art of Walking, The History, Science, Philosophy, and Literature of Pedestrianism*. New York, NY: Riverhead Books.

Pretor-Pinney, G. 2006. *The Cloudspotter's Guide: The Science, History, and Culture of Clouds*. New York, NY: TarcherPerigee.

Armitage, S. 2013. *Walking Home: A Poet's Journey*. New York, NY: Liveright Publishing.

Speck, J. 2013. *Walkable City: How Downtown Can Save America, One Step at a Time*. New York, NY: North Point Press.

APPENDIX

B

Health Questionnaires and Waiver Examples

The following examples are forms that the authors have used in their businesses.

Other options include the following:

- Get Active Questionnaire (GAQ) https://store.csep.ca/products/get-active-questionnaire (Canada)
- American Council on Exercise (ACE) Lifestyle and Health - History Questionnaire https://acewebcontent.azureedge.net/healthcoach resources/pdfs/LifestyleandHealth-HistoryQuestionnaire.pdf

Health and Activity Questionnaire

	YES	NO
Has your doctor ever said that you have a heart condition?		
If yes, please specify:		
Do you feel pain in your chest when you do physical activity?		
If yes, have you spoken with your doctor about this pain?		
If yes, please specify your doctor's diagnosis and recommendations:		
In the past month, have you experienced chest pain when inactive?		
If yes, have you spoken with your doctor about this pain?		
If yes, please specify your doctor's diagnosis and recommendations:		
Do you lose your balance because of dizziness?		
If yes, have you seen your doctor about this condition?		
If yes, please describe your doctor's diagnosis and recommendation:		
Do you ever lose consciousness?		
If yes, have you seen your doctor about this condition?		
If yes, please describe your doctor's diagnosis and recommendations:		
Have you ever experienced a bone or joint injury or illness?		
If yes, please describe:		
Are you currently taking medication for blood pressure or a heart condition?		
If yes, please describe:		

	YES	NO
Do you have any of the following:		
Type I Diabetes (Insulin Dependent)		
Type II Diabetes		
Hypoglycemia		
Multiple Sclerosis		
Osteopenia		
Osteoporosis		

© Lee Scott and Michele Stanten LLC. For reference only, not for reproduction.

Asthma		
Cancer		
Anxiety		
If you answered yes to any of the questions above, please describe your doctor's advice for activity:		
Please describe any past injury, health condition, or experience not listed above that may affect your ability to participate in physical activity:		

I have read, understood, and completed this questionnaire to the best of my knowledge.

NAME (please print): ____________________

SIGNATURE ____________________

DATE ____________________

Health History

1. Name: ____________________

2. Age: __________

3. How would you describe your present state of health?

   ___very healthy
   ___healthy
   ___unhealthy
   ___ill
   ___other
   (please specify: ____________________)

4. Are you taking any prescription medication? If so, what and why?

© Lee Scott and Michele Stanten LLC. For reference only, not for reproduction.

5. Do you take any over-the-counter medication (including vitamins or herbal products)? If so, what and why?
6. When was the last time you visited your physician?
7. Please check any that apply to you and list any important information about your condition:

   ___allergies
   (please specify: ______________________________)
   ___anemia
   ___anxiety
   ___arthritis
   ___asthma
   ___celiac disease
   ___chronic sinus condition
   ___constipation
   ___Crohn's disease
   ___depression
   ___diabetes
   ___diarrhea
   ___disordered eating
   ___food intolerances, e.g., lactose intolerant
   (please specify: ______________________________)
   ___gastroesophageal reflux disease (GERD)
   ___high blood pressure
   ___high cholesterol
   ___hypoglycemia
   ___hypo/hyperthyroidism
   ___insomnia
   ___intestinal problems
   ___irritability
   ___irritable bowel syndrome (IBS)
   ___menopausal symptoms
   ___osteoporosis
   ___premenstrual syndrome (PMS)
   ___polycystic ovary syndrome
   ___pregnant
   ___ulcer
   ___skin problems

© Lee Scott and Michele Stanten LLC. For reference only, not for reproduction.

8. Please list any major surgeries that you've had as an adult.

9. Please list any significant injuries that you've had as an adult.

10. Please describe any other health conditions you may have.

11. Has anyone in your immediate family been diagnosed with any of the following? If so, please list who and at what age they were diagnosed.

    ___heart disease
    ___high cholesterol
    ___high blood pressure
    ___cancer
    ___diabetes
    ___osteoporosis

12. Weight: ____________________

13. Height: ____________________

14. In general, what are your health/fitness goals? What is your motivation to start a walking program?

15. What obstacles do you foresee that may make it difficult for you to walk regularly?

16. Anything else that you'd like for me to know?

Walking and Exercise History

Name: ____

Age: ____

Phone number: _______________________________________

Email: ____

Emergency contact: ___________________________________

Emergency contact phone number: _______________________

© Lee Scott and Michele Stanten LLC. For reference only, not for reproduction.

Please give as much detail as possible.

Are you currently walking for exercise? If yes, how often and for how long do you walk?

Are you currently doing any other types of exercise? If yes, what and how often?

If you are not currently walking/exercising, when was the last time that you did any type of exercise on a regular basis?

Have you ever participated in any type of physical activity events such as 5Ks, marathons, triathlons, etc.? If so, what did you do and when?

What are you hoping to achieve from coaching?

Fitness History and Contact Information

Name: ______________________________

Age (to save me the math): ______________________________

Birthdate (so we can celebrate you!):______________________________

T-shirt size (women's cut): ______________________________

Address:______________________________

Email: ______________________________

Cell #: ______________________________

Emergency contact

(just in case I don't hear from you for a stretch):______________________________

Relationship: ______________________________

Emergency contact cell #: ______________________________

Is it OK if I share your email and/or cell # with the group? __________

Are you interested in receiving reminders via text, email, or both? ___

© Lee Scott and Michele Stanten LLC. For reference only, not for reproduction.

The following information will help me to personalize the experience for you!

Weight (totally confidential, but it will help me to customize the program for you):

Height (without this, the number on the scale is meaningless):

Are you currently exercising (be honest)?

If you are, what are you doing, how frequently are you doing it, how often are you doing it, and for how long have you been doing this? Please include all types of activities and provide the above information for each.

If you are not currently exercising, have you done so in the past?

If you have, what did you do, how frequently did you do it, how often did you do it, for how long had you done it, and when had you done this? Please include all types of activities and provide the above information for each.

Have you even done a 5K, 10K, half marathon, full marathon, triathlon, or other distance event, for example like a fundraising walk? If so, please list what you did, when you did it, and whether or not you walk or ran it. I'd also love to hear if you were happy with your results/experience and why or why not.

Tell me about your motivation for signing up for this. What do you hope to accomplish (aside from crossing the finish line)? Do you want to do it in a particular time? Are you more interested in health or body improvements (be specific)? Want to just start exercising more regularly? Just looking for a fun fitness challenge with friends? Just tell me about your hopes and dreams of what you are expecting from this experience.

In general, what are your health/fitness goals?

What obstacles do you foresee that may make it difficult for you to walk regularly?

Anything else that you'd like for me to know?

© Lee Scott and Michele Stanten LLC. For reference only, not for reproduction.

Waiver Examples

WoW POWER WALKING®
& MORE

WoW Power Walking Waiver

I am participating in this WoW Power Walking course at my own risk and waive all claims of every nature against WoW Company and any coaches on contract with WoW Company and all other associations, sponsoring companies, and sanctioning bodies, in respect to any personal loss or damage, illness, bodily injury, or death resulting from participating in this course and/or activity or caused by third parties during the course and/or activity. I understand the physical risk and rigors associated with power walking and I have prepared myself physically for it. I assume the risk of power walking and walking on or near roads, on sidewalks, in trails and other locations in or out of doors. I hereby grant to WoW Company the exclusive right to free use of my name, voice, and/or picture in any broadcast, telecast, advertising, promotion, website, or other account of the WoW Power Walking programs. By signing below I acknowledge having read, understood and agreed to this waiver and release liability, and understand that I am participating in it at my own risk.

Print name: ______________________________

Signature: ______________________________

Date: ______________________________

Phone: ______________________________

Email: ______________________________

Class location, start date, and time: ______________

If under 18, a parent or guardian must sign.

© Lee Scott and Michele Stanten LLC. For reference only, not for reproduction.

MICHELE STANTEN LLC RELEASE

I, ________________________________, have agreed to voluntarily participate in an exercise program, including, but not limited to aerobic exercise, strength training, and flexibility development, under the guidance of Michele Stanten. I hereby stipulate and agree that I am physically and mentally sound and currently have no physical conditions that would be aggravated by my involvement in an exercise program. I have completed a Get Active Questionnaire and have consulted with a licensed physician, at my discretion.

I understand and am aware that physical-fitness activities, including the use of equipment, are potentially hazardous activities. I am aware that participating in these types of activities, even when completed properly, can be dangerous. I agree to follow the instructions issued by the coach.

Although Michele Stanten will take precautions to ensure my safety, I expressly assume and accept sole responsibility for my safety and for any and all injuries that may occur. In consideration of the acceptance of this entry, I, for myself and for my executors, administrators, and assigns, waive and release any and all claims against Michele Stanten LLC and any of their staffs, officers, officials, volunteers, sponsors, agents, representatives, successors, or assigns and agree to hold them harmless from any claims or losses, including but not limited to claims for negligence for any injuries or expenses that I may incur while exercising or while traveling to and from training sessions. These exculpatory clauses are intended to apply to any and all activities occurring during the time for which I am training with Michele Stanten.

I consent to the use and reuse by Michele Stanten LLC of my name and any images taken during this program in any and all media now known or hereafter devised, worldwide in perpetuity, in or in connection with the training and/or any other Michele Stanten LLC product, program, or service, as well as the promotion, publicity, advertising, and marketing thereof.

I represent and warrant I am signing this agreement freely and willfully and not under fraud or duress.

© Lee Scott and Michele Stanten LLC. For reference only, not for reproduction.

HAVING READ THE ABOVE TERMS AND INTENDING TO BE LEGALLY BOUND HEREBY AND UNDERSTANDING THIS DOCUMENT TO BE A COMPLETE WAIVER AND DISCLAIMER IN FAVOR OF MICHELE STANTEN LLC, I HEREBY AFFIX MY SIGNATURE HERETO.

____

Client's name (please print clearly)

____

Date

____

Client's signature

____

Client's address

© Lee Scott and Michele Stanten LLC. For reference only, not for reproduction.

APPENDIX C

Business Development Resources

Outdoor Session Location Analysis

Are permits necessary? ______________________________

Getting to class and arrival

Commute considerations:

Parking options:

Free: ______________________________

Paid: ______________________________

Public transit:

Accessibility: ______________________________

Time restrictions: ______________________________

Start of class

Storage for valuables: ______________________________

Restrooms: ______________________________

Potable water: ______________________________

During class

Sidewalk safety: ______________________________

Day: ______________________________

Night: ______________________________

Road safety:

Day: ______________________________

Night: ______________________________

Variety of routes:

Trails: ______________________________

Greenspace: ______________________________

Residential: ______________________________

Other: ______________________________

Sidewalks:

Vehicular traffic at intersections: ______________________________

Pedestrian traffic: ______________________________

Visibility: ______________________________

Day: ______________________________

Night: ______________________________

Road shoulders:

Vehicular traffic ______________________________

Pedestrian traffic: ______________________________

Visibility: ______________________________

Day: ______________________________

Night: ______________________________

Winter considerations (e.g., plowed/unplowed, visibility):

Washrooms: ______________________________

Other: ______________________________

Summer considerations (e.g., shade, greenspace, benches):

Washrooms: ______________________________

Other: ______________________________

Pricing Comparison

	Gym name	Annual*	Seasonal	Class pass	Drop-in	Specials**	Payment options	Refund policy
Competitor 1								
Competitor 2								
Competitor 3								
Your business								

*Set an annual percentage increase

**Specials may include season specials, new member specials, customer loyalty specials, early bird options

Administrative Task Management

Task	Frequency	Day/Date/ Time	Assigned to
Renew applicable certifications	Every 2-3 years (confirm with your certification provider)		
Renew CPR/AED and First Aid certifications	Bi-annually		
Renew insurance	Annually		
Plan special events	Annually		
Review collaborations/ community outreach, and location permits	Annually		
Attend a conference	Bi-annually or annually		
Meet with coaches	Semi-annually		
Schedule classes	Quarterly		
Review website	Quarterly		
Update website	Quarterly		
Write and send newsletter	Monthly		
Bookkeeping tasks	Weekly		
Track attendance	Weekly		
Send email to current clients	Weekly		
Plan workouts	Weekly		
Email coaches	Weekly		
Update social media	Daily or every other day		
Personal walk	Daily		
Read	Daily		

Marketing & Promotion Plan for a Class Session

PROGRAM NAME	Details	6 months out	3 months out	6 weeks out
Start date				
Length of session				
Frequency				
Website				
Facebook				
Instagram				
Twitter				
Advertising				
Press releases				

Weekly Class Schedule

Fill in the time, class description, and location for every class you teach. If you have other coaches who lead classes, either fill out a separate schedule for each coach, or use one master schedule and indicate the coach's name for each class.

Time slot	Monday	Tuesday	Wednesday	Thursday	Friday	Saturday	Sunday
Example: 6:30am-7:30am (60 MIN)				*Walking Workout 60 @ The Runner's Shop*			
Example: 7:30am–9:00am (90 MIN)						*Walking Workout 90 @ Sunnybrook Park*	

8-Week Class Plan

List the specific focus, drills, exercises, stretches, or other notes under the headings. Week 1 is filled in as an example.

WEEK 1	WEEK 2	WEEK 3	WEEK 4	WEEK 5	WEEK 6	WEEK 7	WEEK 8
Warm-up	**Warm-up**	**Warm-up**	**Warm-up**	**Warm-up**	**Warm-up**	**Warm-up**	**Warm-up**
Stroll (5 min) Squats, squat with alternating leg abduction, arm circles, calf pumps ~(5 min)							
Go-recover drills	**Go-recover drills**	**Go-recover drills**	**Go-recover drills**	**Go-recover drills**	**Go-recover drills**	**Go-recover drills**	**Go-recover drills**
Basic timed intervals WP<RP (10 min), WP=RP (~10 min)							
Self-compete drills	**Self-compete drills**	**Self-compete drills**	**Self-compete drills**	**Self-compete drills**	**Self-compete drills**	**Self-compete drills**	**Self-compete drills**
Beat the clock 3 reps 30 seconds 3 reps 45 seconds 3 reps 60 seconds (~18 min)							
Strength exercises	**Strength exercises**	**Strength exercises**	**Strength exercises**	**Strength exercises**	**Strength exercises**	**Strength exercises**	**Strength exercises**
2 sets, 12 reps R/L Stationary lunges (~3-5 min)							
Cool-down stretches	**Cool-down stretches**	**Cool-down stretches**	**Cool-down stretches**	**Cool-down stretches**	**Cool-down stretches**	**Cool-down stretches**	**Cool-down stretches**
Stroll (3 min) At wall: gastroc, soleus, hamstring, glute, quad/hip flexors, shin w/o wall, gentle twist (~5-8 min)							

INDEX

ABOUT THE AUTHORS

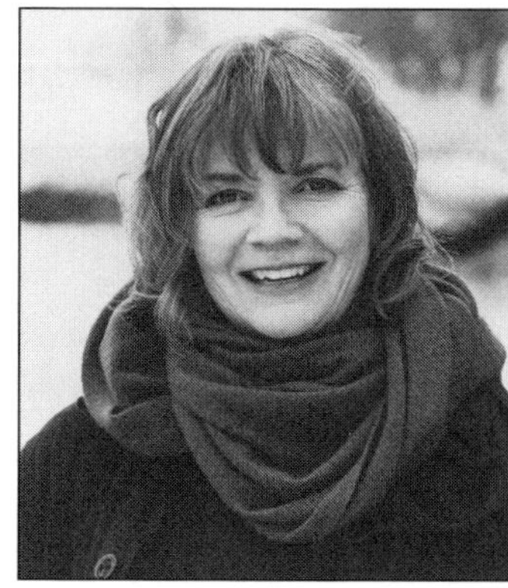

Lee Scott, B.A.Sc., M.A. is an ACE-certified personal trainer and hatha yoga teacher with degrees in mechanical engineering and philosophy of technology.

For almost 30 years, Lee has been bringing a research-based and innovative approach to fitness leadership, with a unique focus on the walking workout. Lee created the WoW Power Walking® program in 2002 and later produced the Simple Secrets for a Great Walking Workout (DVD-CD), offering tips on walking technique and workouts. She has been featured as a walking expert at fitness conferences and race clinics, in magazines, and on television and radio.

Lee has coached thousands of people to bring fresh air, walking, and exertion together in a joyful, accessible, sweaty workout. She has competed in hundreds of distance events including 33 full marathons, consistently winning walk-only competitions since 2002. Lee lives in Toronto, Canada where she enjoys a daily walk no matter what the weather.

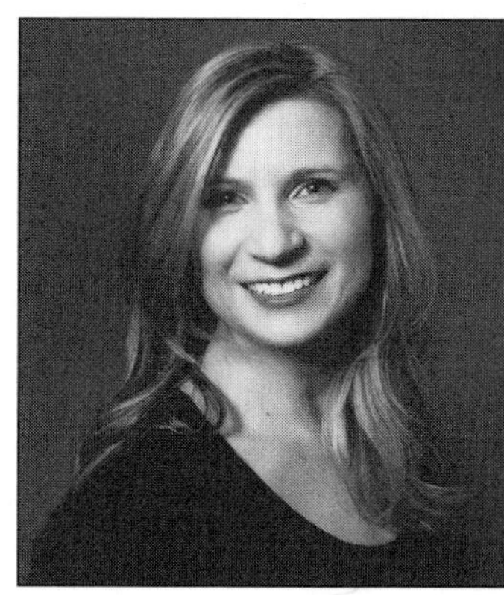

Michele Stanten, a walking coach and ACE-certified fitness instructor, is author of *Walk Off Weight* and creator of mywalkingcoach.com. She's designed walking and fitness programs for leading brands including Harvard Health Publishing, SilverSneakers, Avon, Weight Watchers, and Dr. Oz.

As the former fitness director of *Prevention* magazine, Michele created a marathon walking program and coached thousands of readers to walk full and half marathons across the country. She also helps running events from 5Ks to half marathons to be walker-friendly.

Michele serves on the Every Body Walk! Collaborative coordinating committee and the ACSM Health & Fitness Summit planning committee. She is a past member of American Council on Exercise's Board of Directors. Her many media appearances include The Today Show, Good Morning America, The Dr. Oz Show, The Biggest Loser, CNN, and NPR.

Michele lives in Pennsylvania with her husband, two children, dog, and cat.

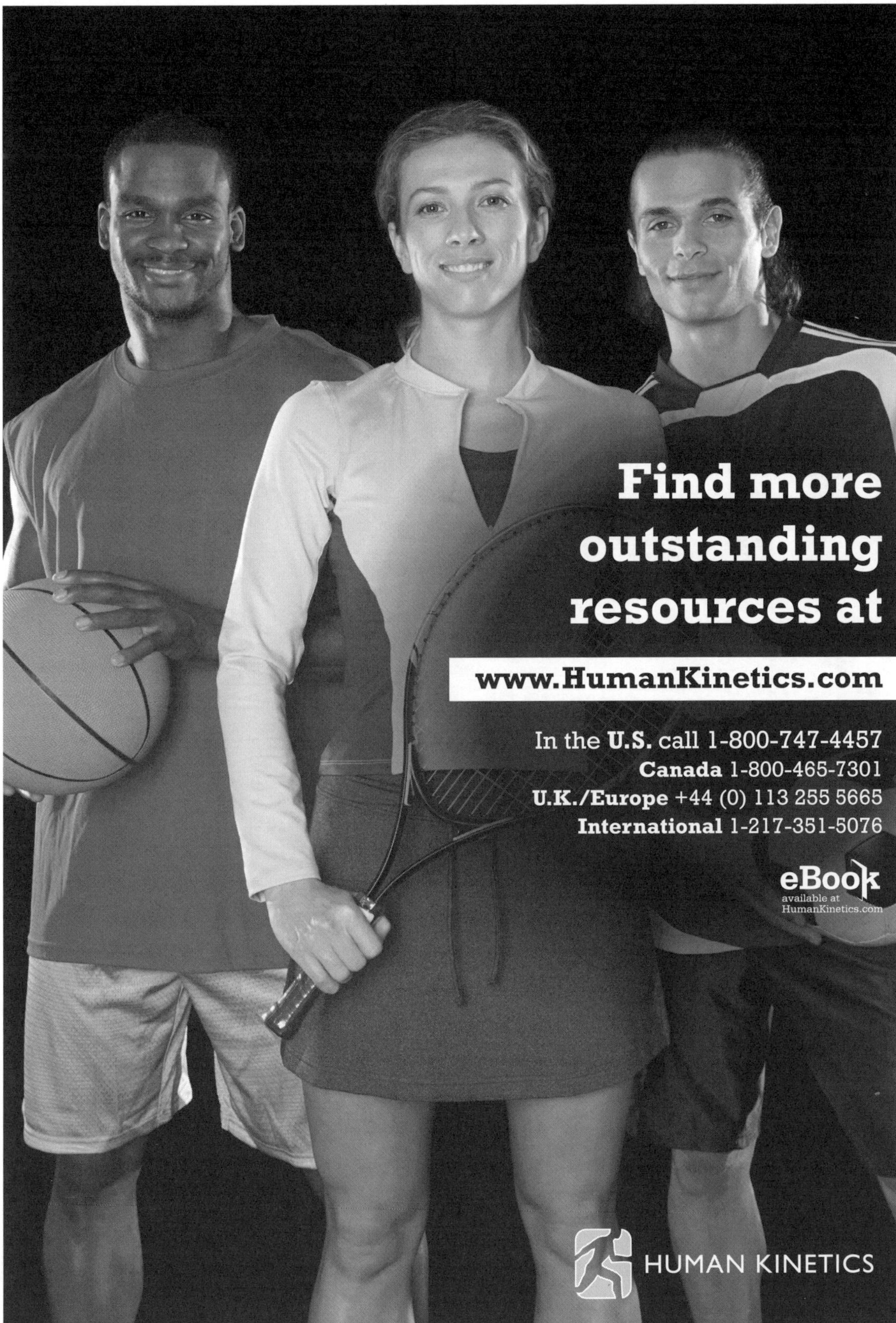
Find more outstanding resources at
www.HumanKinetics.com
In the U.S. call 1-800-747-4457
Canada 1-800-465-7301
U.K./Europe +44 (0) 113 255 5665
International 1-217-351-5076
eBook
available at HumanKinetics.com
HUMAN KINETICS

You read the book—now complete an exam to earn continuing education credit!

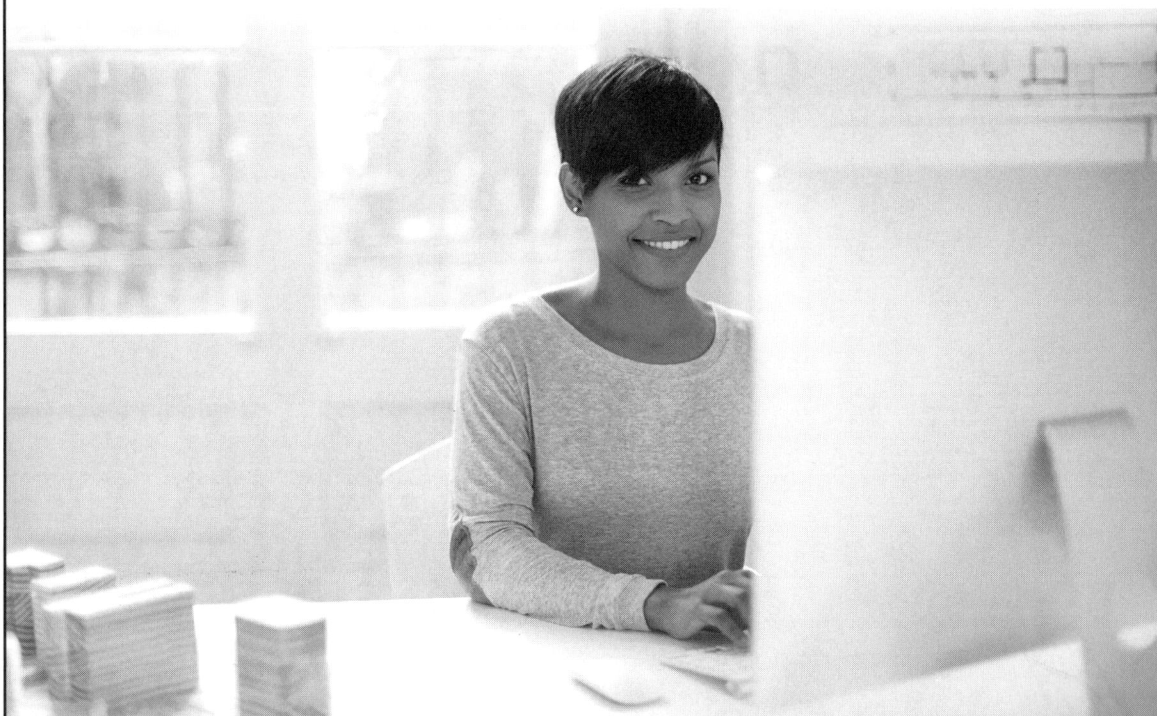

Congratulations on successfully preparing for this continuing education exam!

If you would like to earn CE credit, please visit

www.HumanKinetics.com/CE-Exam-Access

for complete instructions on how to access your exam. Take advantage of a discounted rate by entering promo code **WS2020** when prompted.

HUMAN KINETICS

WS2020

2/19